"I, having lived through rape, and also having raised a child 'conceived in rape,' feel personally assaulted and insulted every time I hear that abortion should be legal because of rape and incest. I feel that we're being used to further the abortion issue, even though we've not been asked to tell *our side* of the story . . ."

-*Kathleen DeZeeuw*
Rape survivor and mother of Patrick

Victims and Victors

*Speaking Out About Their
Pregnancies, Abortions, and Children
Resulting from Sexual Assault*

Edited by

David C. Reardon,

Julie Makimaa,

&

Amy Sobie

Acorn Books
Springfield, IL

Soli Deo Gloria

Dedicated to the brave women
who were willing to share their stories

Victims and Victors: Speaking Out About Their Pregnancies, Abortions, and
Children Resulting from Sexual Assault

Published by Acorn Books, PO Box 7348, Springfield, IL 62791-7348
Printed in Canada

Book and Cover Design: Hunter Design Associates

Portions of this book were originally published in David C. Reardon, *Aborted Women, Silent No More* (Chicago: Loyola University Press, 1986) and *The Post-Abortion Review,* Issue 2(1), Winter 1993.

Cataloging-in-Publication Data
David C. Reardon, Julie Makimaa, and Amy Sobie
    Victims and victors: speaking out about their pregnancies, abortions,
and children resulting from sexual assault / edited by David C.
Reardon, Julie Makimaa, and Amy Sobie
    p.   cm.
Bibliography: (p.   )
Includes bibliographical references.
1. Abortion—United States—Psychological aspects.
2. Abortion—Moral and ethical aspects.
I. Title.
HQ767.4 2000 363.4'6   LCCN: 00-90074
                          CIP
ISBN 0-9648957-1-4

TABLE OF CONTENTS

Section III
Incest And Abortion

Section IV
Finding Better Answers

FOREWORD

Opinion polls show that the vast majority of people accept the "necessity" of abortion in cases of rape and incest. People who oppose abortion in such cases are generally dismissed as heartless extremists.

After all, it is very true that women who become pregnant as a result of rape or incest face extremely difficult circumstances that should invite our compassion and support. To many people, the argument that a woman should not have to spend nine months carrying her attacker's child seems like a natural extension of that compassion.

Sincere empathy for the victims of sexual assault, combined with the widespread confusion, fear, and revulsion associated with rape and incest, made this issue a natural "hard case" for the proponents of legalized abortion. In both Britain and the United States, the legalization of abortion on demand followed public acceptance of abortion as a justifiable "treatment" for rape and incest pregnancies. Once this "exception" was allowed, there was no rational basis for banning abortions in other cases where pregnancy might impose hardship on women.

This was the proverbial "camel's nose" in the tent. It didn't take long for the rest of the camel to follow. What began as social acceptance of abortion in a few rare cases necessarily led to social acceptance of abortion in virtually any circumstance.

Clearly, this is a pivotal issue that pro-life advocates must thoroughly understand if we ever hope to "drive the camel out." But instead, most pro-life activists will continue to squirm and equivocate when asked about abortion for rape or incest pregnancies. Most politicians who have pledged to support a ban on abortion will nonetheless, in submission to the opinion polls, vote to provide public funding for abortions following rape or incest.

All of this is extremely unfortunate because literally *all* of the evidence regarding this issue is on our side. It is a little known fact that the vast majority of sexual assault victims do not want abortions. In addition, when sexual assault victims *do* have abortions, the long term, and even short term, psychological effects are devastating. Most of these women describe the negative effects of abortion on their lives as even more devastating than the sexual assault.

Sexual assault is actually a *contraindication* for abortion. A doctor treating a pregnant sexual assault victim should advise against abortion precisely *because* of the traumatic nature of the pregnancy.

If counselors and physicians truly want to help the victims of sexual assault, they must learn these facts. If pro-life politicians truly want to make a difference, they must learn these facts. If pro-life advocates truly want to restore protection for all unborn children, regardless of how they were conceived, they must learn how to argue on behalf of *both* these unborn children *and* their mothers. If you fit into any of these categories, this book is for you.

More importantly, this book is for the women who have been denied a voice in this debate for far too long: the women who have actually experienced pregnancy following rape or incest.

Please, listen to these women. Learn from them. They will teach you how to be bold in your defense of both them and their children, born and unborn.

It is estimated that rape and incest pregnancies account for only one percent of all abortions. But this one percent is the cornerstone on which tolerance for the other 99 percent of abortions has been built. Moreover, this cornerstone is not strong. It is made of glass, a mirror of our own ignorance and prejudices. It can be broken by giving the women who have been pregnant following sexual assault, whether they carried to term or had an abortion, the chance to have their voices heard.

We have failed to challenge the pro-abortionists' claim that they speak on behalf of these women and their "need" for abortion. You, and every reader of this book, by virtue of your exposure to these testimonies, are being called to correct this oversight.

Challenge them.

Insist that your friends, colleagues, and opponents have an obligation to listen to these women.

Show that you care as much about these women as you do about their children, and that you care far more about *both* than the pro-abortionists who are exploiting them.

We can and we must knock out this cornerstone. Abortion will not end until we dispel confusion by proclaiming the truth—without exceptions.

Section I

Overview and Survey Results

CHAPTER ONE

RAPE, INCEST AND ABORTION: SEARCHING BEYOND THE MYTHS

David C. Reardon, Ph.D.

"How can you deny an abortion to a twelve-year-old girl who is the victim of incest?" complains an angry supporter of abortion. "And how can you call yourself a loving Christian if you would force a victim of violent rape to give birth to a rapist's child?"

Every pro-lifer has heard these same challenges in one form or another. These emotionally charged questions are usually used in an attempt to prove that pro-lifers are either 1) insensitive "fetus lovers" who don't care about women, or 2) ethically inconsistent, allowing abortion for some circumstances but not for others.

Unfortunately, most pro-lifers have difficulty answering these challenges because the issue is so widely misunderstood. Typically, both sides of the debate accept the presumption that most women who become pregnant following sexual assault want abortions. From this "fact," it naturally follows that the reason women want abortions in these cases is because it will help them to put the assault behind them, recover more quickly, and avoid the additional "trauma" of giving birth to a "rapist's child."

But in fact, the welfare of a mother and her child are never at odds, even in sexual assault cases. As the testimonies in this book confirm, both the mother and the child are helped by *preserving* life, not by perpetuating violence. Sadly, however, the testimonies of women who have actually been pregnant through sexual assault are routinely left out of this public debate. Most people, including sexual assault victims who have never been pregnant, are therefore forming opinions based on their own prejudices and fears rather than the real life experiences of those people who have been in this difficult situation and reality.

For example, it is commonly assumed that rape victims who

become pregnant would naturally want abortions. But in the only major study of pregnant rape victims ever done prior to this book, Dr. Sandra Mahkorn found that 75 to 85 percent chose *against* abortion. This figure is remarkably similar to the 73 percent birth rate found in our sample of 164 pregnant rape victims. This one finding alone should cause people to pause and reflect on the presumption that abortion is wanted or even best for sexual assault victims.

Several reasons are given for not aborting. First, approximately 70 percent of all women believe abortion is immoral, even though many also feel it should be a legal choice for others. Approximately the same percentage of pregnant rape victims believe abortion would be a further act of violence perpetrated against their bodies and their children.

Second, many of these women believe that their children's lives may have some intrinsic meaning or purpose which they do not yet understand. This child was brought into their lives by a horrible, repulsive act. But perhaps God, or fate, will use the child for some greater purpose. Good can come from evil.

Third, victims of assault often become introspective. Their sense of the value of life and respect for others is heightened. Since they have been victimized, the thought that they in turn might victimize their own innocent children through abortion is repulsive.

Fourth, the victim may sense, at least at a subconscious level, that if she can get through the pregnancy she will have conquered the rape. By giving birth, she can reclaim some of her lost self-esteem. Giving birth, especially when conception was not desired, is a totally selfless act, a generous act, a display of courage, strength, and honor. It is proof that she is better than the rapist. While he was selfish, she can be generous. While he destroyed, she can nurture.

ADDING FUEL TO THE FIRE

If giving birth builds self respect, what about abortion? This is a question which most people fail to even consider. Instead, most people assume that abortion will at least help a rape victim put the assault behind her and get on with her life. But in jumping to this conclusion, the public has adopted an unrealistic view of abortion.

Abortion is not some magical surgery which turns back the clock to make a woman "un-pregnant." Instead, it is a real life event which is always very stressful and often traumatic. Once we accept that abortion is itself an event with deep ramifications on a woman's life, then we must look carefully at the special circumstances of the pregnant sexual assault victim. Will having an abortion truly console her, or will it only cause further injury to her already bruised psyche?

In answering this question, it is helpful to begin by noting that many women report that their abortions felt like a degrading form of "medical rape." This association between abortion and rape is not hard to understand.

Abortion involves a painful intrusion into a woman's sexual organs by a masked stranger who is invading her body. Once she is on the operating table, she loses control over her body. If she protests and asks the abortionist to stop, chances are she will be either ignored or told: "It's too late to change your mind. This is what you wanted. We have to finish now." And while she lies there tense and helpless, the life hidden within her is literally sucked out of her womb. In both sexual and medical rape, a woman is violated and robbed. In the case of sexual rape she is robbed of her purity. In the case of medical rape via abortion, she is robbed of her maternity.

For many women this experiential association between abortion and sexual assault is very strong. It is especially strong for women who have a prior history of sexual assault, whether or not the aborted child was conceived during an act of assault. This is just one reason why women with a history of sexual assault are likely to experience greater distress during and after an abortion than are other women.

Second, research shows that after any abortion, it is common for women to experience guilt, depression, feelings of being "dirty," resentment of men, and lowered self-esteem. These feelings are identical to what women typically feel after rape. Abortion, then, only adds to and accentuates the traumatic feelings associated with sexual assault. Rather than easing the psychological burdens of the sexual assault victim, abortion adds to them.

This was the experience of Jackie Bakker, who reports: "I soon discovered that the aftermath of my abortion continued a long time after the memory of my rape had faded. I felt empty and horrible. Nobody told me about the pain I would feel deep within causing nightmares and deep depressions. They had all told me that after the abortion I could continue my life as if nothing had happened."[1]

Those encouraging abortion often do so because they are uncomfortable dealing with sexual assault victims, or perhaps because they harbor some prejudice against victims whom they feel "let it happen." Wiping out the pregnancy is a way of hiding the problem. It is a "quick and easy" way to avoid dealing with the woman's true emotional, social and financial needs.

Kathleen DeZeeuw, whose son Patrick was conceived in rape when she was 16, writes,

> I, having lived through rape, and also having raised a child 'conceived in rape,' feel personally assaulted and insulted every time I hear that abortion should be legal because of rape and incest. I feel that we're being used by pro-abortionists to further the abortion issue, even though we've not been asked to tell our side of the story.

TRAPPING THE INCEST VICTIM

The case against abortion for incest pregnancies is even stronger. Studies show that incest victims rarely ever voluntarily agree to abortion. Instead of viewing the pregnancy as unwanted, the incest victim is more likely to see the pregnancy as a way out of the incestuous relationship because the birth of her child will expose the sexual activity. She is also likely to see in her pregnancy the hope of bearing a child with whom she can establish a truly loving relationship, one far different than the exploitive relationship in which she has been trapped.

But while the incest victim may treasure her pregnancy because it offers her the hope of release from her situation, it poses a threat to the man who is exploiting her. It is also poses a threat to the pathological secrecy which may envelop other members of the family who are afraid to acknowledge the abuse. Because of this dual threat, the victim may be coerced into an unwanted abortion by both the abuser and other family members.

For example, Edith Young, a 12-year-old victim of incest impregnated by her stepfather, writes twenty-five years after the abortion of her child:

Throughout the years I have been depressed, suicidal, furious, outraged, lonely, and have felt a sense of loss . . . The abortion which was to 'be in my best interest' just has not been. As far as I can tell, it only 'saved their reputations,' 'solved their problems,' and 'allowed their lives to go merrily on.' . . . My daughter, how I miss her so. I miss her regardless of the reason for her conception.

Abortion providers who routinely ignore this evidence and neglect to interview minors presented for abortion for signs of coercion or incest are actually contributing to the victimization of young girls. Not only are they robbing the victim of her child, they are concealing a crime, abetting a perpetrator, and handing the victim back to her abuser so that the exploitation can continue.

Finally, we must recognize that children conceived through sexual assault also deserve to have their voices heard. Rebecca Wasser-Kiessling, who was conceived in a rape, is rightfully proud of her mother's courage and generosity and wisely reminds us of a fundamental truth that transcends biological paternity: "I believe that God rewarded my birth mother for the suffering she endured, and that I am a gift to her. The serial rapist is not my creator; God is."

Similarly, Julie Makimaa, who works diligently against the perception that abortion is acceptable or even necessary in cases of sexual assault, proclaims, "It doesn't matter how I began. What matters is who I will become."

That's a slogan we can all live with.

NOTES

1. David C. Reardon, *Aborted Women, Silent No More* (Chicago, IL: Loyola University Press, 1987), 206.

CHAPTER TWO

A SURVEY OF RAPE AND INCEST PREGNANCIES

Amy Sobie & David C. Reardon

The testimonies used in this book were gathered from 192 women who became pregnant as a result of rape or incest and from 55 children conceived in sexual assault. These testimonies were collected over a nine-year period by Fortress International and the Elliot Institute.

Some of the respondents filled out detailed surveys. Others submitted letters or testimonies that were not specifically structured for data gathering. While an effort was made to have all the respondents fill out a survey in order to obtain the most information possible, some respondents did not complete or return the lengthy form. Many of our requests for additional information were returned with notices that their forwarding address information had expired. In these cases, the original contact letters we received from these women were the only information we had for the contextual analysis provided below.

Many of the original contact letters were quite expansive and addressed most of the questions raised in the survey. In a few cases, however, we were only able to extract a few points of information, such as the outcome of the pregnancy, but not details about the emotional impact of that experience.

The testimonies collected represent a very diverse sample of sexual assault experiences. In some cases, women wrote about sexual assault pregnancies that had taken place many years before, while for others, the sexual assaults had occurred just a few years or even months before. Two of the women were pregnant from sexual assault at the time they responded to the survey. And while most of the women had achieved at least some measure of peace and healing from these past events, others—especially those who for whom the emotional scars were most recent—were still trying to painfully reconcile their experiences.

There were also 55 responses from children who had been conceived in rape or incest, most of whom are now adults. Some of these children were raised by their birth mothers; others were placed for adoption.

It is worth noting that we also received letters from parents, relatives, and friends of sexual assault survivors. In addition, we received about a dozen letters from parents who adopted children conceived in rape or incest. While none of these testimonies were included in the book or in the following analysis, they were helpful in providing a broader understanding of these issues.

An Overview of the Data

Of the 192 women who had become pregnant through sexual assault, 164 had been victims of rape, while 28 were victims of incest (sexual assault involving a family member). Of these, 69 percent chose to carry their pregnancies to term, 29 percent had abortions, and 1.5 percent had miscarriages.

Of the 164 women who became pregnant as the result of rape, 73 percent carried the pregnancy to term, 26 percent had abortions, and 2 percent had miscarriages. Of the 119 women who carried the pregnancy to term, 36 percent chose to place their children for adoption, while 64 percent retained custody of their children. One of these women who carried to term also reported five pregnancies resulting from the incest/rape of her adoptive father, all of which were miscarried.

Of the 28 women who became pregnant as the result of incest, 50 percent carried the pregnancy to term and 50 percent had abortions. One young woman gave birth to two children fathered by her father. The first was raised in the family, while the second was placed for adoption. Of the other thirteen women who gave birth, the children of five were placed for adoption, and the remaining eight were raised by the birth mother, a family member, or a combination thereof.

Women Who Had Abortions

Of the 56 women who had abortions, six did not provide any information on how they felt about their abortions.

Of the remaining 50, only one rape victim reported no regrets about her decision to abort. One incest victim stated that she felt abortion was the correct choice in her case, but she did not comment about whether or not it had affected her. Four indicated numerous regrets related to the abortion but were ambivalent about whether or not it was the right choice. Their responses might be characterized by, "It bothers me a lot but maybe it was for the best. There are good things about my life now which maybe I wouldn't have if I had the baby." Forty-four women (88 percent of those expressing an opinion on their abortions) explicitly regretted their abortions and stated that it had been the wrong solution to their pregnancies.

Among the 44 victims of rape who aborted, 30 expressed an opinion as to whether or not abortion was an appropriate solution to offer women who become pregnant from rape. Of these, twenty-eight (93 percent) said their abortions had not been a good solution to their problems and stated that they would not recommend it to others in their situation. Only two women (7 percent) supported the view that abortion was "usually" a good solution in such cases. Of these two, only one said she had no regrets about her own decision to abort. In this case, her pregnancy and abortion had been recent events.

It is notable that 19 of the 44 rape victims who aborted (43 percent) indicated that they felt pressured or strongly directed by family or health care workers to choose an abortion. For these women, the desire to abort did not originate from within themselves, but was instead a concession to the suggestions or demands of others. Following are some examples from their testimonies:

> I was 22 weeks pregnant and had decided I really wanted to keep my baby. But I felt a tremendous pressure from all sides—especially to please my parents—and I finally gave in.

> My mom told me abortion was the only answer and I was such an emotional wreck that I just thought if that's what she thinks, she must be right. So that day she took me and paid for my abortion.

> My parents were embarrassed about the pregnancy and insisted I have an abortion . . .

> I went in for "counseling" beforehand . . . When I look back, she [the counselor] was more of a salesperson than a counselor. I mentioned all of my doubts about the abortion and she would try to tear them down.

[My] pastor was very non-judgmental. I wanted him to tell me that abortion was wrong. He didn't really tell me anything . . . I did not have the support I needed to make the decision.

The doctor advised me to have an abortion. Since abortions were illegal at the time I would not have considered that as an available option, but the doctor gave me the name of a respected doctor in his medical building who routinely did abortions . . .

I went to Rape Crisis and they offered to pay for the abortion. There was no alternative from them, the clinic, or even the few friends who knew [about the rape]. I chose abortion thinking it was really the only solution.

Basically my friend took me by the hand and led me to the clinic where there was no discussion about alternatives, just an appointment made for me . . .

Of the 14 incest victims who had abortions, eleven explicitly stated that abortion was not a good solution and they would not recommend it to others. Of the remaining three, one woman expressed the idea that abortion had not been a good decision in her case, but she did not address the issue in regard to other women. The second woman was "uncertain" if abortion was the right solution for others and gave no indication of how it had affected her. Only one woman said that abortion was "usually" the solution to rape and incest pregnancies, but she did not indicate whether or not she had experienced any emotional effects from her abortion.

In almost every case where an incest victim had an abortion, it was the girl's parents or the perpetrator who made the decision and arrangements for the abortion, not the victim herself. None of these women reported having any input into the decision. Each was simply expected to comply with the choice of others. In several cases, the abortion was carried out over the objections of the girl who clearly told others that she wanted to give birth to her child. In a few cases, as in the example of Edith Young's testimony, the victim was not even clearly aware that she was pregnant or that she was undergoing an abortion.

In sum, nearly all of the sexual assault victims who had undergone abortions report that the abortion only compounded their problems, and that they regret having had the abortion. Of those who expressed an opinion, over 90 percent stated that they would discourage other sexual assault victims from having an abortion. Only three supported the view that abortion is usually a good solution to sexual assault pregnancies.

WOMEN WHO CARRIED TO TERM

In our contextual analysis of the testimonies and letters from the 133 women who carried to term, over 80 percent explicitly expressed happiness that they had chosen to give birth to their child. *None* of the women stated that they did not want their child or a wish that they had chosen abortion instead.

Of the 119 rape victims who carried the pregnancy to term, 25 women did not express their feelings about the pregnancy, their child, or the idea of abortion. Instead their initial contact letters focused on the trauma of sexual abuse and what they had done to find healing.

Of the 94 remaining women, all expressed satisfaction with their decision to have the baby. Most stated that they had not considered abortion to be a good solution for them and/or that they had turned down a suggestion that they abort. Many had withstood tremendous pressure from family, friends, or medical personnel to have an abortion.

Of the 82 women who expressed an opinion about abortion, 77 (94 percent) rejected the idea of abortion as a good option for pregnancies resulting from sexual assault. Of the remaining five, one was uncertain how she would advise another woman. The other four, while happy that they had chosen to have their babies, expressed the view that abortion "might" be okay in some cases or that women should be free to make their own choice.

Of the 14 incest victims who carried the pregnancy to term, all were happy that they had been able to carry to term. Of these women, five did not express an opinion regarding abortion. The other nine unanimously rejected abortion as a good option for incest-related pregnancies.

Notably, *not one* of the 133 women who carried their pregnancies to term expressed regret over having given birth to their children, or a wish that they had chosen abortion instead. This includes women who were still struggling with the trauma of sexual assault, and also a few women who had chosen to raise their children themselves but, in retrospect, believed *adoption* might have been a better option for them and their children.

Finally, there were three women in the survey whose pregnancies ended in miscarriage or "spontaneous abortion." Of these women, two were pro-life and intended to carry the pregnancy to term (although one stated that she prayed for a miscarriage.) One of these women had a positive first pregnancy test, while a later test came up negative, indicating that she might not have actually been pregnant. The intentions of the third woman were unknown.

CHILDREN CONCEIVED IN SEXUAL ASSAULT

As mentioned above, we collected letters and testimonies from 55 children who had been conceived in sexual assault. These respondents ranged in age from teenagers to adults. Some had been raised by their birth mothers, while others had been placed for adoption. Of those placed for adoption, many had been reunited with their birth mothers and had learned about their conceptions from them.

Obviously, none of the children who responded expressed the view that they wished their mothers had aborted them. Whether raised by their birth mothers or placed for adoption, most reported that they had happy, healthy, productive, normal lives. Many also expressed indignation or even anger at the idea that they were somehow "products of evil" or that anyone conceived as they were should be aborted.

From their letters, it was clear that most of the children had a healthy acceptance of the knowledge that they had been conceived in sexual assault. Some had found this acceptance more difficult to achieve than others, and some who had only recently learned of the circumstances of their conception were still struggling to integrate this knowledge into their view of themselves and of the world around them. Most of the writers expressed great gratitude to their mothers for choosing to give them life, often in the face of social or familial pressure to abort.

The overwhelming theme of the children's letters was that they deserved to live, regardless of the circumstances of their conception. In addition, they did not believe that the circumstances of their origins should be seen as a handicap or an impediment to their lives in any way.

SELECTION OF TESTIMONIES

In choosing the testimonies to be reprinted in this book, the editors attempted to use those testimonies that were the most detailed, articulate, and broadly representative of the experiences and views of the women and children in each category.

SECTION II

RAPE AND ABORTION

CHAPTER THREE

HOW ABORTIONISTS HAVE EXPLOITED THE VICTIMS OF RAPE

David C. Reardon, Ph.D.

Rape is a powerful word. It elicits feelings of both sympathy and horror. People readily sympathize with rape victims, but they also recoil from thinking too deeply about the experience of rape. This results in a curious mixture of both immediate empathy and deep-seated ignorance, a combination that has made rape an extremely useful tool for advancing the agenda of abortion on demand.

Before abortion was legal, abortion advocates focused their initial efforts on this "hard case" issue. "Should a woman who is pregnant from rape be *forced* to carry the child of her brutal attacker?" they asked. It is difficult for anyone to answer "yes" to such a question. (In many cases, the question was also posed with an appeal to racial prejudices: "Would you oppose an abortion if your daughter was raped by a black man?")

Through such appeals, abortion advocates won public support for at least a few abortions in such "hard cases." Laws were changed. The unborn child's right to life was no longer considered sacred or fundamental. But once any exception to the general prohibition on abortion was made, logic demanded that this exception should be expanded into a general license for abortion on demand. After all, if a woman should not be "forced" to carry the child of an unwanted rape, on what grounds could she be "forced" to carry the child of any unwanted father?

The confusion arising from the rape exception played readily into the hands of those whose real goal was abortion on demand. For example, does the rape exception include "statutory rape," where any minor under the age of 17 is considered "raped" whether she agreed to intercourse or not? Does the rape have to have been reported? Can a woman claim the right to abortion if she only reports the rape after she confirms that she is pregnant, even months after the incident?

In fact, to require the woman to report the rape is patently uncompassionate and unrealistic. Many rape victims are so terrified and emotionally bruised by the experience that they do not report the rape and cannot, as a rule, be expected to do so.

Once the emotional wedge of the rape "exception" was pushed into abortion legislation, other restrictions on abortion completely lost their moral imperative. If we allow abortion when a man forces himself upon a woman, then it seems to follow that we should allow abortion when an unborn child "forces" himself or herself upon the woman.

It was exactly this logic that prevailed in *Doe v. Bolton*, the companion case to the better known *Roe v. Wade*. In *Doe*, the Supreme Court struck down a Georgia law which prohibited abortion except in cases of rape. The Court ruled that by allowing abortion in *some* cases, the state was admitting that the unborn child's right to life was not absolute. If abortion was allowed in cases of rape, there was no justifiable reason for the State to "arbitrarily" forbid abortion under other compelling circumstances.

Abortion proponents have skillfully used the public's sympathy for rape victims and the ambiguities surrounding rape to convince the public that at least some abortions are justified. They claim that the issues are too complex to understand, much less restrict through legislation. Therefore, they argue, it is best to leave the abortion decision to women and their physicians.

While the pro-abortion rape argument has been effective, it has unfortunately proven to be a grave disservice to both women in general and pregnant rape victims in particular. As we shall see, while claiming to speak on behalf of pregnant rape victims, abortion advocates have routinely ignored their real needs and the trauma abortion causes to these women. Their argument for abortion in these "hard cases" is not only shallow and paternalistic, it is also exploitive.

The public has uncritically accepted the claim that abortion is the "best" way to help pregnant rape victims escape the burden of bearing "a rapist's child." The evidence, however, is to the contrary.

THE PSYCHOLOGY OF RAPE VICTIMS

Rape is a deeply traumatic experience which results in "guilt, anger, fear and a myriad of other, often overpowering, emotions [which] require ventilation."[1] The trauma of rape can cause or aggravate psychological disorders.

One psychological condition frequently associated with rape is post-traumatic stress disorder (PTSD). PTSD is a psychological illness which results from a traumatic experience that overwhelms and distorts a person's normal defense mechanisms. The victim experiences such deep shock that his or her emotional defenses become disorganized and disconnected from reality, either temporarily or for a prolonged, indefinite period of time.

Any event that arouses intense feelings of fear, helplessness, or loss of control may be traumatic. A diagnosis of PTSD requires identification of symptoms in three categories: hyperarousal, intrusion, and constriction.

Hyperarousal is a characteristic of inappropriately and chronically aroused "fight or flight" defense mechanisms. In some way, the person is almost always "on the alert" for threats of danger. Symptoms of hyperarousal include exaggerated startle responses, anxiety attacks, difficulty falling asleep or staying asleep, irritability, outbursts of anger or rage, aggressive behavior, difficulty concentrating, hypervigilence, or physiological reactions upon exposure to situations that symbolize or resemble an aspect of the traumatic experience. As an example of the latter, a woman traumatized by rape (or abortion) may break into a sweat or experience an elevated pulse during a routine pelvic exam.

Intrusion is the reexperience of the traumatic event at unexpected times. Symptoms of intrusion include recurrent and intrusive thoughts, flashbacks, or nightmares about the traumatic event.

Constriction is the numbing of one's emotions or the development of behavior patterns designed to avoid any sights, sounds, smells, or feelings associated with the trauma. This may include the inability to recall aspects of the traumatic experience; efforts to avoid activities, situations, places or people associated with the traumatic event; a more restricted range of emotions; a sense of a foreshortened future (e.g., the victim does not expect to have a career, marriage, children, or a long life); diminished interest in previously enjoyed activities; drug or alcohol abuse; suicidal thoughts or acts; and other self-destructive tendencies.

The experience of all three types of reactions after a trauma (hyperarousal, intrusion, and constriction) is a sign that the person's normal defense mechanisms have taken on a life of their own. They are governing emotions or behavior in inappropriate ways. As a result, the victim may develop abnormal behaviors or even major personality disorders.

For example, some PTSD victims may experience intense emotions but have no clear memory of the event, while others may remember every detail but feel no emotion. Still others may reexperience both the event and the emotions in intrusive and overwhelming flashbacks that are emotionally devastating.

Any traumatic experiences, such as witnessing a violent crime, being in combat, or even being in a car accident, can result in PTSD. The experience of rape is even more complicated than the "typical" traumatic experience, since it includes additional layers of social, moral, and psychological issues related to self-esteem. (This is also true in the case of abortion, as we shall see.)

One of the complicating factors is that victims of rape often feel that they are suspected by others of either lying about the attack or are guilty of having invited or allowed it to happen. The victim's fear of judgment by family, friends, or society in general is a major factor in why so many rapes are unreported. The perceived attitude of those around them is also related to the sense of shame and self-reproach which women feel toward themselves.

This self-blame also contributes to unreported rapes. "Believing that she is somehow tainted, dirty, and dehumanized, and knowing that many will view her either as pitiful and helpless or as disgusting and defiled, she [the rape victim] often takes great pains to conceal the fact of the assault."[2]

The social issues surrounding rape can severely inhibit emotional recovery following rape. For example, even simple questions from family, friends, or police can inadvertently aggravate feelings of self-reproach. The question, "Why did you go there with him?" will be interpreted as, "Why did you put yourself into such a dangerous situation?" Asking, "Did you scream?" implicitly questions whether the victim struggled hard enough to resist the attack.

For both the victim and her loved ones, the question "Why did this happen to me/her?" is critical, perplexing and troubling. Recovery from a traumatic experience demands an effort to understand what has happened. But in asking the questions that lead to understanding, one faces moments of self-doubt and self-blame.

These issues are aggravated by the widely held view that "nice girls don't get raped." This prejudice suggests that if a woman is raped, she is not or never was a "nice girl." Thus, any questions as to why the attack happened, by others and even by herself, can ultimately reinforce feelings of guilt, shame, and self-blame: "Despite its irrationality a sense of guilt is common, a consuming search for some flaw or characteristic which has caused the victimization. Anger, finding no legitimate outlet, may be turned inward, being nurtured by self-blame and often released as self-punishment."[3]

Both the victim and her loved ones may find that the search for understanding is like walking through a mine field. But standing still is not much better. This happens when friends and family feel so uncomfortable or embarrassed about the incident that they take great pains to avoid discussing it or to conceal the tragedy. Such "brush it under the rug" attitudes may only end up making the victim feel more isolated and alone. "Often relatives and friends try to dissuade her from thinking or talking about it (the assault) in the mistaken belief that she will become more emotionally distressed. However, if others refuse to listen, the patient [who has been raped] may conclude that they are embarrassed and ashamed and want to punish her for what has happened."[4]

In addition, because rape involves a sexual act, the victim will often feel "defiled" or "tainted." If she is married, her spouse may also struggle with this issue. In fact, the rapist has indeed intruded onto the sacred ground of their private sexual relationship, and the memory of the rape can for a time haunt their sexual relationship. It is not unusual for the woman and her husband to face struggles in putting the rape behind them.

For these reasons, proper care for rape victims should include counseling not only for the victim, but also for her friends and family. This task becomes even more important in the rare cases where pregnancy results, or when there is even the suspicion of a rape pregnancy.[5]

THE EXTRA PREJUDICES SURROUNDING RAPE VICTIMS WHO BECOME PREGNANT

Besides dealing with all the "normal" trauma associated with rape, the pregnant woman faces additional pressures because of her pregnancy. The social attitude that rejects the victim as "unclean" also rejects the "tainted" offspring who is the evidence of the crime. This deep-seated prejudice is revealed in the tendency to refer to the baby as the "rapist's child" rather than the woman's child.[6]

These prejudices tend to lump the child into the same category as the rapist—to view him or her as an evil or criminal entity. A rape pregnancy is seen as the result of "ugly" or "sinful" sex, so the child is automatically seen as "ugly" or "sinful." The idea of the child as a separate, innocent person, as a lovable new baby, is easily lost among the heavy, entangling prejudices surrounding rape and rape victims. To a society squeamish about rape, a pregnancy resulting from sexual assault signifies "only a blot to be removed."[7]

These public and personal prejudices are deeply ingrained. Rape is an uncomfortable issue. Few people know how to sensitively deal with rape victims, much less *pregnant* rape victims. When faced with discomfort and confusion, we latch on to myths, prejudices, and slogans. Abortion seems like a quick, easy, and attractive solution.

From this viewpoint, it is clear that abortion in these cases is convenient chiefly for society, which is already predisposed to reject the rape victim. Indeed, it is quite telling that the leading organizations that promote abortion using the rape and incest argument have *never* sought the opinions of the pregnant sexual assault victims themselves. They have never surveyed their needs. Instead, they have simply *presumed* that a pregnant rape victim would want an abortion, would need an abortion, and would benefit from an abortion. They are content with this presumption because it (1) fits our social prejudices about rape and incest and (2) advances the political agenda for abortion on demand.

STUDIES OF THE EMOTIONAL ADJUSTMENTS OF WOMEN MADE PREGNANT THROUGH RAPE

Few researchers have studied the psychology of pregnant rape victims. Prior to this book, the only published research on this topic was that of Dr. Sandra Mahkorn, an experienced rape counselor who first published a report on her research in 1979. In studying the case histories of 37 pregnant rape victims who had been counseled by various social welfare agencies, Dr. Mahkorn found that 28 women chose to continue their pregnancies, five chose abortion, and the outcome for the remaining four could not be determined. This finding—that between 75 and 85 percent of pregnant rape victims actually choose *against* abortion—clearly contradicted the assumption that most rape victims want abortions.[8]

Among those who refused abortion, most took the view that abortion was simply another act of violence, that it was immoral, or that it was killing. One woman expressed the belief that she "would suffer more mental anguish from taking the life of the unborn child than carrying the baby to term." Others felt that the child had an intrinsic meaning or purpose, making statements such as: "All life has meaning," or, "This child can bring love and happiness into someone's life."

Of the 28 who carried their children to term, Mahkorn found that 17 chose adoption, three chose to keep the child, and details for the remaining eight were unknown.

Most of the women stated that their primary problem was the need to confront and deal with "feelings or issues related to the rape experience," although a significant minority (19 percent) placed primary emphasis on the need to confront and explore feelings about the pregnancy, including feelings of "resentment," "hostility toward the child," and "denial of the . . . pregnancy."[9]

When asked what conditions or situations made it most difficult for them to continue the pregnancy, most women responded that it was social pressure—the opinions, attitudes, and beliefs of others about the rape and pregnancy. Reasons included "family pressure [to abort]," "attitudes of boyfriends," and the belief that "people will not believe that she was raped or that it could have been prevented." Such feelings of rejection because she is "unclean" increase the victim's own sense of self-rejection and compel her to "cover up" what has happened. Under such pressure, abortion may seem the only solution because it will conceal the crime and "cleanse" the woman of rape's stains.

Rejection of the victim and suspicions about her culpability may increase among her family and friends when the pregnancy is discovered. Their discomfort around the rape victim increases, because the pregnancy itself becomes a permanent symbol of the rape, a constant reminder of her defilement—at least until it is aborted. In Jackie Bakker's case, she reported that

"When I learned I was pregnant, my boyfriend and all my friends—including [my girlfriend who was with me when we were raped that night]—deserted me. They all acted like I was the 'plague.'"

Though some women initially felt angry with the unborn child because of the attack, Mahkorn found that these women consistently had more positive attitudes as the pregnancy progressed. The overwhelming majority of the women had a better self-image and a positive view of the child by the time of delivery. None of the women displayed more negative attitudes, a fact which prompted Dr. Mahkorn to write:

> The belief that pregnancy following rape will emotionally and psychologically devastate the victim reflects the common misconception that women are helpless creatures who must be protected from the harsh realities of the world . . . [This study illustrates] that pregnancy need not impede the victim's resolution of the trauma; rather, with loving support, nonjudgmental attitudes, and empathic communication, healthy emotional and psychological responses are possible despite the added burden of pregnancy.[10]

Rape counselor Joan Kemp also reports that this pattern of initial negative feelings toward the child followed by a growing sense of acceptance is quite normal:

> After sexual assault there is, for varying lengths of time, a natural revulsion toward anything associated with the rape. They may include the location, or characteristics of the rapist such as his clothing, race, mustache, etc. It is normal for this feeling to attach to the unborn child conceived in rape. However, these feelings normally fade with time. When this does not happen spontaneously, counseling with someone qualified to treat victims of trauma is highly effective. Rape victims I have worked with were quite aware and distressed by the inappropriateness of these feelings. They would not, for instance, have welcomed anyone telling them that men of their attacker's race are natural criminals. Nor do women welcome being told that their children conceived in rape are unworthy of life, genetically prone to crime, and bound to feel unwanted and bitter. *A person in crisis is seeking positive solutions, not a counsel of despair.*[11]

The fact that women who bear children conceived in rape learn to treasure their children is so evident that even a reporter for the pro-choice *Glamour* magazine could not escape this conclusion. After interviewing women and their adult children conceived in rape, the writer felt compelled to state as one of her primary conclusions that "It is a stunning fact of these stories that in each case, the mother was able to overcome her loathing for her rapist and instead find joy in her love for her child."[12]

Dr. Mahkorn's study led her to conclude that encouraging abortion as the solution to a rape pregnancy is, in fact, counter-productive, because abortion only reinforces *negative* attitudes. Her observations are worth quoting at length:

> Because it is likely that the victim already harbors feelings of guilt as a result of the assault, medico-social pressures which encourage and result in abortion could compound the woman's feelings of guilt and self-blame [over the abortion itself] . . . Perhaps as a result of their own biases and an unwillingness to deal with the more emotionally difficult complications of a pregnant rape victim, many physicians suggest abortion in this case as one would prescribe aspirin for a tension headache . . . While on the surface this 'suggestion' may appear acceptable and even 'humane' to many, the victim is dealt another disservice. Such condescending ['quick-fix'] attitudes on the part of physicians, friends and family can only serve to reaffirm the sense of helplessness and vulnerability that was so violently conveyed in the act of sexual assault itself. At a time when she is struggling to regain her sense of self-esteem, such a 'take charge' attitude can be especially damaging. Often the offer of such 'quick and easy' solutions as abortion only serves those who are uncomfortable or unwilling to deal with the special problems and needs that such complications as pregnancy might present.
>
> . . .The central issue, then, should not be whether we can abort all pregnant sexual assault victims, but rather an exploration of the things we can change in ourselves, and through community education, to support such women through their pregnancies. The 'abortion is the best solution' approach can only serve to encourage the belief that sexual assault is something for which the victim must bear shame—a sin to be carefully concealed . . . too often the pregnancy receives the most attention and the anger, guilt, fear, and lower self-esteem related to the assault fail to be addressed.
>
> . . . [The] attitudes projected by others and not the pregnancy itself pose the central problem for the pregnant victim.
>
> By no means am I attempting to conclude that pregnancy as a result of rape is a simple matter. Such a conclusion would indeed be naive. This study does seem to suggest, however, that even though emotionally and psychologically difficult, these burdens

can be lessened with proper support.[13] [Emphasis added]

ABORTION AS ANOTHER SEXUAL ASSAULT

"Rape" and "abortion" are both harsh, cruel words. They are words which provoke such revulsion that people don't like to think about either the acts or the victims involved. The world would no doubt be better without both rape and abortion, but unfortunately people are afraid to confront either. It is better, somehow, to try to ignore them, put them out of mind, and pretend that they never happen.

Given such a widespread denial of reality, it is not surprising that abortion is unlikely to relieve the rape victim's anxieties. Instead it is much more likely to add to and complicate her emotional trauma.

Even researchers who support abortion on demand have confirmed that sexual assault is a "predictor" of post-abortion trauma. For example, mental health researcher Gloria Zakus reports:

> Certain categories of women are much more likely to have post-abortion problems sometimes months or years later . . . Women with a history of sexual abuse, including incest, molestation, or rape, may respond with great anxiety to abortion plans, encompassing even the initial pelvic exam. On a conscious or unconscious level, these women may associate gynecological and abortion procedures with previous aggressive violations. One such case involving a teenager in an incestuous relationship with her father required hospitalization and the use of a general anesthetic in order to do a suction procedure.[14]

Even post-abortion women who have not been sexually assaulted occasionally describe the experience of abortion as "surgical rape."[15] This analogy is not surprising when one considers the actual mechanics of abortion. The woman is prone on her back, legs spread, with a masked stranger plunging instruments into her sexual organs, painfully and literally sucking life out of her womb. This symbolic reenactment of the rape can hardly be lost on the victim of sexual assault who is still struggling for recovery.

"Linda" described her abortion as follows:

> I was fully awake, no pills given, or shots. I lay there with tears rolling down my face. The room was cool. My tears felt like fire

on my face, cutting it, slice by slice, tear by tear. My hands were
wet with sweat, my right hand squeezed the counselor's thin,
cold hand as though squeezing the life out of her. My left hand
lay fisted, clenched tightly on my vibrating stomach as the abortion occurred. It felt as though someone was raping me with a
15-amp canister vacuum hose with no mercy as I lay there helpless, crying calmly, as if agreeing to be raped.

The similarities between abortion and rape are more than
superficial, however. The emotional impacts of these traumas
are, in fact, identical in many respects.

Like rape, abortion causes feelings of guilt, lowered self-
esteem, feelings of being sexually violated, feelings of having
lost control or of being controlled by circumstances, suspicion of
males, sexual coldness, and most of the other symptoms related
to post-rape trauma. For pregnant rape victims, abortion tends
only to accentuate and reinforce the negative feelings caused by
rape. Abortion doubles the impact of these negative feelings
while doing nothing to promote the inner healing which is so
desperately needed.

As previously mentioned, rape can frequently result in post-
traumatic stress disorder. Abortion, also, can cause PTSD.[16] An
important study of women who had abortions three years previously found that one of every five women who had an abortion suffered from diagnosable PTSD. Approximately half had
many, but not all, the symptoms of PTSD, and 20 to 40 percent
showed moderate to high levels of stress and avoidance behavior relative to their abortion experiences.[17]

Since abortion can cause PTSD, it should be immediately evident that abortion is actually a contraindication for rape pregnancies, since it is likely to exacerbate, not diminish, the psychological symptoms associated with PTSD.

THE RISK-LADEN DECISION TO ABORT

The women who participated in our study confirm the reports
of therapists that the negative feelings arising from abortion
after rape are often worse and more difficult to resolve than the
negative feelings resulting from the rape itself. This is principal-
ly because the woman feels greater responsibility for the abortion than for the rape. This was well expressed by rape victim
"Patricia Ryan," who wrote:

I was an innocent victim of a horrible crime. I was not to blame
for what the rapist did to me. But in choosing to abort, to kill the
innocent child growing within me, I lowered myself to the level
of the rapist . . . It only compounded my pain; it didn't solve anything.

A woman is at risk for suffering long-term mental health
problems after an abortion if any of the following apply to her:
ambivalence or uncertainty about the decision; feeling pressured to have an abortion; adolescence or immaturity; prior
emotional or psychiatric problems; prior low self-image; prior
children; a prior abortion; religious or conservative values; a
desire to keep the abortion a secret; lack of support from their
partner; lack of support from their parents; abortion of a
planned child due to fetal abnormalities; a second or third
trimester abortion; or a history of sexual assault.[18]

It is especially useful to take a closer look at the first two of
these general high-risk criteria: ambivalence about the decision
and feeling pressured to have an abortion.

Public opinion polls show that approximately 70 percent of
women believe abortion is immoral, or the taking of a life,
although many may support the right of others to choose abortion.[19] This figure almost exactly matches research results taken
at abortion clinics, which have found that 70 percent of women
having abortions actually have a negative moral view of abortion.[20] Most of these women have abortions not because they
believe it is all right to do so, but because they feel that given
their circumstances, they have no other choice.[21]

These studies also show that more than half of post-aborted
women report feeling "forced" to have an abortion by others. In
one study, 84 percent stated they would have carried the pregnancy to term under "better circumstances."[22] Thus, for such a
high risk patient, abortion is not an exercise of freedom and liberation, but instead a capitulation to outside pressures which
"force" her to violate her own conscience.

Many women have described their abortion decision as an
"evil necessity" to which they submitted because they "had no
choice." Afterwards they were plagued by a sense of self-betray-
al. One woman described herself as a "spineless coward."
Another said that all the abortion did for her was to reveal "how
evil I can really be."[23]

By failing to stand up for what she truly believes in her heart,
such a high-risk woman feels that she has betrayed both herself

and her child. She is internally divided by an emotional "war" within and against herself. On one side are her original moral beliefs and maternal desires. On the other side is her abortion experience, which represents a choice to act against those feelings. These two sides of herself are irreconcilable.

This internal warfare can destroy a woman's self image and manifest itself in a wide variety of psychological illnesses, including drug and alcohol abuse, suicidal behavior, emotional numbness, emotional breakdown, radical personality changes, memory loss, sleep disorders, sexual dysfunction, increased tendency toward violence, child abuse, difficulty bonding with later children, psychosomatic illnesses, and more.[24]

RISKS WITHOUT BENEFIT

Even in more general terms, all the available research unanimously shows that the existence of any psychological problems prior to an abortion reliably predicts greater psychological problems after an abortion. In other words, prior emotional problems (including a history of trauma) are a *contraindication* for abortion, since the pre-existing emotional problems are generally complicated and aggravated by abortion rather than alleviated.[25] Indeed, there is not even *one* psychiatric condition for which abortion is a recognized cure or a beneficial treatment.[26] Nor are there any statistically-validated studies that support the view that abortion produces any lasting benefit to women's emotional or physical health in any general circumstance, much less in the specific case of traumatic rape.

Besides these psychological risks, abortion poses significant risks to a woman's reproductive health. These risks include infection and cervical damage, which can lead to sterility; increased rates of miscarriage, premature labor, and ectopic pregnancies; labor complications in subsequent deliveries; subsequent children suffering death or neonatal handicaps related to premature birth; breast cancer; cervical cancer; and maternal death related directly to the abortion or to subsequent reproductive health problems. The risk of suffering from any of these complications is increased if the woman is an adolescent or undergoes more than one abortion.[27]

Victims of sexual assault who have abortions are not spared these psychological and physical risks. Indeed, as discussed earlier, they are at an even higher risk than the "normal" population of experiencing psychological complications that are created or aggravated by the abortion.

Given that (1) abortion involves a large number of well documented physical and psychological risks, and (2) there is no medical evidence that abortion is actually beneficial in any general or particular circumstance, it is clear that there is no reasonable medical basis for recommending or performing abortions. This is especially true in cases where the patient has pre-existing risk factors that increase the likelihood that she will experience negative reactions, such as pregnancy resulting from sexual assault. All the presumed benefits of abortion in this case are simply and only that—presumed, in spite of all the evidence to the contrary.

MIXED UP FEARS, MIXED UP CHOICES

Proponents of abortion claim that abortion for the pregnant sexual assault victim will somehow benefit her psychological recovery. But they offer no evidence to support this claim. Indeed, as discussed above, all the existing documentation based on interviews with women who have actually been in this situation contradict this claim.

Pro-abortionists also suggest that women who are pregnant from sexual assault want to have abortions. Again, this presumption is offered without any supporting documentation and is contradicted by the findings of two independent studies (Mahkorn's and ours) that the majority of women pregnant from rape actually choose to carry to term.

Despite all this evidence to the contrary, the pro-abortion presumption that abortion is a necessary "cure" for rape pregnancies is widely accepted by the general public. Why? Because fear creates confusion.

Public support for abortion in cases of rape is rooted in one thing, the abhorrent fear of being raped. The opinion that "I would never want to have a rapist's baby" arises directly from the underlying fear, "I would never want to be raped."

Of course you wouldn't. No one wants to be raped. So it naturally follows that no one would *want* to conceive a baby while being raped.

Indeed, none of the women whose testimonies we gathered

wanted to be raped. Given a choice, none of them would have chosen this way to become pregnant. Before their own experience with rape pregnancies, most would have accepted the idea that abortion might be good in the case of rape pregnancies. It is only when they were actually faced with such a pregnancy that they could see through this universal fear.

The fact that this nearly universal opinion arises purely from fear is demonstrated by this simple observation: while no one wants to be raped, many people do want to have babies. Once this fact is clarified it is obvious that having a baby is not the underlying source of this universal revulsion toward rape pregnancies—it is the fear of rape.

This understanding may also explain why the majority of pregnant rape victims actually choose to carry to term. Prior to their own rape pregnancies, many of these women had opinions that were typical of the general population. Most would have accepted abortion in cases of rape. But after their fears were actually realized, perhaps it was only then that they could they truly see and understand the source of their fear. Only then did it become clear that it was not their unborn children whom they feared, it was the men who had raped them. Once the focus of their fear was clear, the option of abortion, which they had previously imagined as an obvious or easy solution to such a problem, no longer appeared so attractive.

We must remember that these women are not victims of pregnancy. They are victims of *rape*. As will be seen in the following testimonies, the problems of pregnant rape victims "stem more from the trauma of rape rather than from the pregnancy itself."[28] The pregnancy is not a minor issue, but it is still not the cause their trauma.

In these cases, as in every case of an unplanned pregnancy, abortion proponents have confused the issue by describing a woman's choice as simply that of choosing between having a baby or not having a baby. This description is a deceptive oversimplification of the real question facing women.

Abortion is not simply the absence of a child. It not some magical event that simply turns back time so that the woman's life is exactly as it was before the child was conceived.

Once a woman is pregnant, the choice she actually faces is the choice of having a baby or having an abortion—a traumatic experience with physical, psychological, social, familial, and spiritual consequences. Either choice will forever change the woman's life. The suggestion that having an abortion will not affect her life, but will instead return it to the way it was before she became pregnant, is a gross lie.

Abortion not only destroys the life of a woman's unborn child, it also become a permanent part of who she is. The memory of the abortion and of her unborn child becomes a permanent part of her past and her perception of herself. It is a life-changing experience, as significant as any birth or death experience.

Women who have aborted children conceived in rape have consistently reported that abortion did not make their lives better. Instead, it almost always aggravated their emotional suffering and in many cases, also resulted in physical complications.

Conversely, pregnant rape victims who chose to give their children life overwhelmingly report that the choice to give birth was a choice to triumph over the rape. It was a choice which said: "This rape will not dictate my life." It was a choice which wrestled good from evil. Instead of remembering only their fear and shame, these women are now able to remember their strength, courage, and generosity in a time of trial.

Aggravating the Problem

Abortion proponents believe that abortion can solve both individual and social problems. It was once claimed that abortion of "unwanted" children would help to reduce child abuse. Unfortunately, it has had the opposite effect. A history of abortion is associated with an increased risk of child abuse against subsequent "wanted" children.[29]

Similarly, abortion has been proposed as a solution to rape pregnancies, but there is no evidence that the incidence of these pregnancies has declined. Instead, it would appear to be that since the legalization of abortion the incidence of rape has increased, which would also suggest that the total number of rape pregnancies that occur each year is also higher than prior to 1973, when abortion was legalized. While it would be difficult to prove any causal relationship, a reasonable argument can be made to suggest that legalization of abortion may have indirectly contributed to the increased rate of sexual assault, and therefore, an increase in sexual assault pregnancies.

There are several ways in which this may be true. As the

"backup" for failed contraceptive practices, abortion has reduced personal accountability for the procreative aspects of sex. By clearing the path for the "sex is for fun" mentality, abortion has made sexual adventurism more socially acceptable. This in turn has encouraged more eroticism in all forms of the arts and media and a corresponding increase in the number of men exposed to pornographic and sadomasochistic sexual images. This eroticized culture encourages men to believe that they "need" or "deserve" to have sex. This alone may have a direct relationship to the increased incidence of date rapes. In addition, however, the sexual revolution has exacted a terrible emotional price on both women and men. As the last two generations of men have become more sexually promiscuous, they have suffered from the emotional injuries of failed relationships, exaggerated expectations of themselves and women, rejection of their sexual advances, and the loss of their children to both divorce and abortion. Any and all of these experiences can increase the level of anger men feel toward women.

Given these factors, it would not be surprising to find that many men are resorting to rape as a means of acting out their anger toward women. Through acts of sexual assault, they may be expressing an aspect of their own confusion, pain, loss, and anger specifically related to their own sexual experiences.

If this is true even to a small degree, easy access to abortion would exacerbate this problem. Abortion not only encourages sexual irresponsibility among males, it also creates in men feelings of guilt and grief that are, at least in some cases, channeled into anger toward women.[30]

In addition, abortion reflects the view that personal problems can be solved through acts of violence. After all, if a pregnant woman's "needs" are more important than her duty to respect her unborn child's body, why shouldn't a man's "need" for sex or for displays of subservience be more important than his duty to respect his wife, his girlfriend, or a stranger on the street?

Clearly, the problem of rape pregnancies has not been solved by legalizing abortion. Nor has making abortion legal improved the way men treat women. Instead, it is more likely that the opposite is true. Legalized abortion may have actually have contributed to the increase in cases of rape and rape-related pregnancies.

Showing True Compassion for Pregnant Sexual Assault Victims

Clearly, abortion does nothing to alleviate the trauma of pregnant sexual assault victims. At best, it only hides a physical symptom of the rape and spares family members the difficulty of adjusting to the needs of the woman and her child.

As is evident in the testimonies presented in this book, many of the pregnant rape victim's problems stem from society's abhorrence of her condition. Revulsion toward the rape is carried over to both the woman and her child. But are the woman and her child truly tainted by rape? Or is society tainted by superstition and prejudice? If, as we believe, the latter is true, then the cure is not to be found in abortion, but rather in acceptance.

Dr. Mahkorn writes: "Perhaps true liberation for the rape victim means the freedom to publicly acknowledge what has happened without fear of rejection. Perhaps true liberation means the freedom to carry a pregnancy to term with the realization that, like herself, the child is an innocent victim."[31]

Feminist Mary Meehan agrees: "Psychological support, especially from the woman's family and friends, is enormously important. They should stand by her and say clearly that, no matter what the circumstances of conception, there should *never* be any embarrassment about bringing a child into the world. There should never be anything but pride in that."[32]

It is irrational and dangerous for society to make the children conceived in rape the targets of social revenge. These children have done no wrong, and abortion certainly does not undo their fathers' crimes nor mend their mothers' wounds.

Nowhere would the old proverb, "two wrongs don't make a right," seem more appropriate. Even convicted rapists are not punished by execution. Does it make sense that the innocent child should be condemned to death in the father's place?

Does it make sense to heap violence on top of violence, especially when the woman's body and psyche are made the battleground for both attacks? Does it make sense to encourage a victim of violence to find comfort in participating in another violent act?

The public attitude that abortion will somehow "fix" a pregnant rape victim clearly adds to the pressure on sexual assault victims to give in to an unwanted abortion. Hearing the same solution offered by counselors, doctors, family and friends may cause a woman to doubt her own instincts and values. If she follows their uninformed advice, she will only feel betrayed by her advisers when she subsequently learns that the abortion did not solve her problems, but instead made them worse.

"Vanessa Landry," a victim of rape who was coerced into an unwanted abortion, writes:

> People think that whenever anyone is raped, they have to have an abortion. My social worker just kept telling me all kinds of things to encourage me to have an abortion . . . They didn't give me any other option except to abort. They said that if I went on to have the baby I wouldn't have any way of supporting it . . .
>
> I didn't really want to have the abortion. I have always been against abortion all my life. But the doctors told me that if I went on and had the baby, I would die since I'm diabetic, and I believed them. The social workers and my doctor told me all this stuff, you know, that the baby wouldn't be normal, and it would be retarded and deformed . . . Since then I've learned none of this is true . . . Lots of women with diabetes and high blood pressure give birth to normal children . . . Women who are raped can give their babies up for adoption . . .
>
> The doctor and social worker who led me to have the abortion shouldn't have. I would rather have gone on and had the child anyway on my own account. But they pressured me into the abortion, saying that welfare wouldn't pay for giving birth but would pay for the abortion, since they were saying I would die. They said I was just another minority bringing a child into the world and there are too many already.
>
> [After the abortion], I had a lot of bleeding for two or three weeks. I couldn't get over it. I suffered a lot of mental anguish. Every time I see somebody with a little baby, I want to go over and hold it. I very much want to have children.
>
> I'm over the rape now, but because of the abortion I'm not able to have any kids . . . Instead of helping me, all they wanted was to prevent the baby.[33]

Vanessa was exploited not only because she was a rape victim, but also because she was black and poor. Like almost every other victim in our records who aborted a pregnancy resulting from rape, she reports that the negative results of the abortion have lasted far longer than the trauma of the rape.

It is no wonder, then, that women who have been pregnant

through sexual assault are angered by pro-abortionists who exploit their situations for their own political advantage. Kathleen DeZeeuw, whose complete testimony appears later in this book, writes:

> To me, it is an affront every time I hear all the rhetoric from the pro-abortionists. As I stated before, a woman is most vulnerable at a time such as this, and doesn't need to be pounced on by yet another act of violence. She needs someone to truly listen to her, care for her, and give her *time* to heal.
>
> I, having lived through rape, and also having raised a child 'conceived in rape,' feel personally assaulted and insulted every time I hear that abortion should be legal because of rape and incest. I feel that we're being used to further the abortion issue, even though we've not been asked to tell our side of the story.

In light of all this evidence *against* abortion of rape pregnancies, and in the absence of any evidence other than prejudicial opinions *for* abortion, we must ask whether any informed, conscientious physician would ever recommend abortion for a rape pregnancy? Certainly not. He would recognize that what the woman really needs is emotional support and healing from the rape. He would recognize that her confidence and sense of self-worth need to be rebuilt, not destroyed by the added emotional pain of abortion.

At the beginning of this chapter, I asserted that the question, "Should a woman who is pregnant from rape be *forced* to carry the child of her brutal attacker?" is a ploy which preys on social prejudices about rape. The question demands a "no" in the name of compassion, but it is a false compassion, a quick fix, a cheap solution which leaves the woman scarred both by her rape and by her abortion.

I would argue that the real question society must ask itself is this: "Should a woman and her child who is conceived by rape be *abandoned* to care for themselves without the love and support of family, friends, and society?"

This question also demands a "no" answer. But in this form it is a demand for authentic compassion. It demands personal involvement and personal sacrifice on the parts of family, friends, and society so that we might truly help and support victims of sexual assault and their children. This is not the easiest alternative, but it is the only right alternative.

Portions of this chapter were previously published in Aborted Women, Silent No More *by David C. Reardon, Loyola University Press, 1987.*

NOTES

1. Sandra Kathleen Mahkorn, M.D. and William V. Dolan, M.D., "Sexual Assault and Pregnancy," in Thomas Hilgers, Dennis Horan, and David Mall, *New Perspectives on Human Abortion* (Frederick, MD: University Publications of America, 1981), 191.

2. Ibid., 182.

3. Ibid., 185.

4. Sandra Kathleen Mahkorn, "Pregnancy and Sexual Assault," *The Psychological Aspects of Abortion*, David Mall and Walter Watts, eds (Washington D.C.: University Publications of America, 1979), 66.

5. It is likely that many "rape" pregnancies are in fact the result of sexual intercourse between women and their husbands or boyfriends which occurred shortly before the attack. Though the child, in such cases, is not actually the "rapist's," the victim's genuine belief that it is, or may be, causes the same psychological distress as would be faced in any true rape pregnancy. Because such cases are psychologically and emotionally indistinguishable, the need for compassionate treatment is still imperative. See Mahkorn, "Pregnancy and Sexual Assault," 65.

6. Joan Kemp, "Abortion: The Second Rape," *SisterLife*, Winter 1990, Feminists For Life of America, 811 E. 47th St., Kansas City, MO 64110.

7. Mary Meehan, "Accepting the Unjust," *The National Catholic Register*, 18 April 1982.

8. A national survey of adult women regarding sexual assault experiences found that of 3,031 adult women, 413 women reported experiencing 616 rape or incest incidents at some time in their lives, as a result of which 19 women became pregnant, with one woman reporting two such pregnancies. Relying on a variety of polls and national statistics, the authors estimate that based on the result of this random poll, there may be as many as 32,000 pregnancies related to rape or incest each year. Using a slightly larger sample, of which the above women were a subset, the authors also reported that of 30 women reporting 34 sexual assault pregnancies, approximately 50 percent had induced abortions, 6 percent placed the child for adoption, 32 percent were raised by the mother, and 12 percent ended in spontaneous miscarriages.

Approximately 48 percent of these 34 sexual assault pregnancies cases occurred in women between 12 and 17 years of age. In 18 percent of these cases, the perpetrator was identified as a relative, step-father, or biological father. Husbands were identified as the perpetrator in 18 percent of the cases, and boyfriends, friends, or other known persons (non-relatives) accounted for 53 percent of these sexual assault pregnancies. Only nine percent of these cases involved a stranger. Given the small sample sizes involved, these results are not substantially different than the results reported by Mahkorn or in our survey.

Unfortunately, the authors did not report, or perhaps did not undertake, any evaluation by the women of how the experience of pregnancy, childbirth, abortion, or miscarriage had effected the women. Nor did they evaluate the influence of others in the choice to abort or carry to term, which is especially problematic since half of these women were minors and may have been offered little or no choice but an abortion.

Melisa M. Holmes, et.al., "Rape-Related Pregnancies: Estimates and Descriptive Characteristics from a National Study of Women," *Am J Obstet Gynecol* 175(2): 320-324, August 1996.

9. Mahkorn, "Pregnancy and Sexual Assault," 58-59.

10. Mahkorn and Dolan, "Sexual Assault and Pregnancy," 194.

11. Kemp, "Abortion: The Second Rape," op. cit.

12. Jennifer Braunschweiger, "My Father Was a Rapist," *Glamour*, Aug 1999, 251.

13. Mahkorn, "Pregnancy and Sexual Assault," 65-69.

14. Gloria Zakus and Sandra Wilday, "Adolescent Abortion Option," *Social Work in Health Care*, 12(4), Summer 1987, 86-87.

15. Linda Bird Francke, *The Ambivalence of Abortion* (New York: Random House, 1978) 84-95, 167; David C. Reardon, *Aborted Women, Silent No More* (Chicago: Loyola University Press, 1987), 51, 126.

16. Anne C. Speckhard and Vincent M. Rue, "Postabortion Syndrome: An Emerging Public Health Concern," *Journal of Social Issues*, 48(3):95-119 (1992).

17. Catherine A. Barnard, *The Long-Term Psychosocial Effects of Abortion* (Portsmouth, NH: Institute for Pregnancy Loss, 1990).

18. Vincent Rue, Institute for Abortion Recovery and Research, "Pro-Abortion Counseling for Post-Aborted Women: The Implications," 1991 paper session of the Association for Interdisciplinary Research; Senay, "Therapeutic Abortion: Clinical Aspects", *Archives of Gen. Psych.*, 23: 408-415; Friedman, et.al.,"The Decision-Making Process and the Outcome of Therapeutic Abortion," *Am. J. Psychiatry*, v.131, 1332-1337 (1974); Lazarus, "Psychiatric Sequelae of Legalized Elective First Trimester Abortion," *J. of Psychosomatic Ob&Gyn*, 4: 141-150 (1985); Pare and Raven, "Follow-up of Patients Referred for Termination of Pregnancy," *The Lancet*, v.1, 635-638 (1970); Reardon, *Aborted Women, Silent No More*, 131-38.

19. *Los Angeles Times* Poll, March 19, 1989; James Davison Hunter, *Before the Shooting Begins: Searching for Democracy in America's Cultural War* (New York: The Free Press, 1994), 108.

20. Mary K. Zimmerman, *Passages Through Abortion* (New York: Praeger Publishers, 1977), 69, 110-112, 193; Reardon, *Aborted Women, Silent No More*, 11-13; Howard and Joy Osofsky, eds., *The Abortion Experience* (New York: Harper and Row Publishers, Inc., 1973), 196-198.

21. In one poll, 74 percent of women who had a history of abortion agreed with the statement: "I personally feel that abortion is morally wrong, but I also feel that whether or not to have an abortion is a decision that has to be made by every woman for herself." (*Los Angeles Times* Poll, March 19, 1989. See also Reardon, *Aborted Women, Silent No More.*)

22. Reardon, *Aborted Women, Silent No More*, 12.

23. Excerpts from over 2000 first hand accounts of women who have had abortions collected by the Elliot Institute as part of our Case Study Project.

24. Thomas Strahan, *Major Articles and Books Concerning the Detrimental Effects of Abortion: An Annotated Bibliography* (Charlottesville, VA: The Rutherford Institute, 1997), contains the most extensive collection of findings published in the journals of medicine and psychology. See also Reardon, *Aborted Women, Silent No More,* and David C. Reardon, "Psychological Reactions Reported after Abortion," *The Post-Abortion Review* 2(3):4-8, Fall 1994, which contains the summary results of a survey of 260 women who were questioned regarding over a hundred reactions related to abortion. This study, along with numerous other articles and studies regarding the aftereffects of abortion are posted on the Internet at www.afterabortion.org.

25. The following are just a few of many studies linking one or more pre-existing psychological problems with an increased risk of more severe psychological reactions to abortion. J.R. Ashton, "The Psychosocial Outcome of Induced Abortion," *Brit. J. Obstetrics & Gynaecology,* 87: 1115 (1980); Catherine A. Barnard, *The Long-Term Psychological Effects of Abortion* (Institute for Pregnancy Loss, Portsmouth, N.H., 1990); Elizabeth M. Belsey et al., "Predictive Factors in Emotional Response to Abortion: King's Termination Study - IV," *Soc. Sci. & Med.* 11:71 (1977); Council on Scientific Affairs, American Medical Association, "Induced Termination of Pregnancy Before and After Roe v. Wade: Trends in the Mortality and Morbidity of Women," *JAMA* 268:3231 (1992); Cornelia Morrison Friedman, et al., "The Decision-Making Process and the Outcome of Therapeutic Abortion," *Am. J. Psychiatry* 131:1332 (1974); Warren M. Hern, *Abortion Practice* (Boulder, CO: Alpenglo Graphics, Inc., 1990); Bryan Lask, "Short-term Psychiatric Sequelae to Therapeutic Termination of Pregnancy," *Brit. J. Psychiatry* 126:173 (1975); Arthur Lazarus & Roy Stern, "Psychiatric Aspects of Pregnancy Termination," *Clinics Obstetrics & Gynaecology* 13:125 (1986); Warren B. Miller, "An Empirical Study of the Psychological Antecedents and Consequences of Induced Abortion," *J. Soc. Issues* 48(3):67 (1992); Warren B. Miller et al., "Testing a Model of the Psychological Consequences of Abortion, in *The New Civil War: The Psychology, Culture, and Politics of Abortion* (Linda J. Beckman & S. Marie Harvey eds., American Psychological Association, 1st ed. 1998), 235

26. The evidence against abortion as an aid in treating emotional or

psychological problems is compelling, universal, and undisputed. According to Dr. Fred E. Mecklenburg, Professor of Obstetrics and Gynecology at the University of Minnesota Medical School and member of the American Association of Planned Parenthood Physicians:

"There are no known psychiatric diseases which can be cured by abortion. In addition there are none which can be predictably improved by abortion . . . . [Instead,] it may leave unresolved conflicts coupled with guilt and added depression which may be more harmful than the continuation of the pregnancy.

"Furthermore, there is good evidence to suggest that serious mental disorders arise following abortions more often in women with real psychiatric problems. Paradoxically, the very women for whom legal abortion may seem most justifiable are also the ones for whom the risk is highest for post-abortion psychic insufficiency . . . .

"When abortion is substituted for adequate psychiatric care—and there is ample evidence to suggest that this is already happening—then there is a distinct danger of minimizing established psychotherapeutic principles. Unfortunately, it is the distressed woman who ultimately faces the dulling impact of this minimization. She is the one who cries for help and she is also the one who is turned away. " [Fred E. Mecklenburg, M.D., "The Indications For Induced Abortion," *Abortion and Social Justice,* Thomas W. Hilgers and Dennis J. Horan, eds. (New York: Sheed and Ward, 1972), 40.]

Similarly, an official statement from the World Health Organization states: "Thus the very women for whom legal abortion is considered justified on psychiatric grounds are the ones who have the highest risk of post-abortion psychiatric disorders." (Dr. & Mrs. J.C. Willke, *Handbook on Abortion,* Hayes Publishing Co., Inc., 1979, 52)

And an article in the *World Medical Journal* observes that: "[Abortion] is a bad way of treating true psychiatric disease . . . . Investigation shows that there is less psychological trauma associated with normal birth than there is with a legal abortion." (M. Harry, "A Critical Evaluation of Legal Abortion," *World Medical Journal,* 23(6):83-85, 1976).

Many of the mental health care professionals who advocate abortion have admitted that these abortions do not promote medical or psychological welfare, but insisted that they are "therapeutic" in a sociologic way because they prevent "unwanted" children. In 1971, for example, Dr. Seymour Halleck, a Wisconsin psychiatrist, wrote:

"No psychiatrist, if he is honest with himself . . . can . . . describe any scientific criteria that enable him to know which woman should have her pregnancy terminated, and which should not. When he recommends an abortion, he usually lies. It is a kind lie, a dishonesty intended to make the world a little better, but it is still a lie." (James Tunstead Burtchaell, *Rachel Weeping,* Kansas City: Andrews and McMeel, Inc., 1982, 69.)

At worst, abortion is recommended by mental health workers

because a pregnant patient increases the work load of the staff at psychiatric hospitals. (See Reardon, *Aborted Women, Silent No More*,169-170.)

27. Reardon, *Aborted Women, Silent No More*, 89-114; Strahan, *Major Articles and Books Concerning the Detrimental Effects of Abortion: An Annotated Bibliography*, 95-122; Ann Saltenberger, *Every Woman Has a Right to Know the Dangers of Legal Abortion* (Glassboro, NJ: Air-Plus Enterprises, 1982), 55-135.

28. Mahkorn and Dolan, "Sexual Assault and Pregnancy," 190.

29. Ney, P., Fung, T., Wickett, A.R., "Relationship Between Induced Abortion and Child Abuse and Neglect: Four Studies," *Pre- and Perinatal Psychology Journal* 8(1):43-63, Fall 1993; Benedict, M., White, R., and Cornely, P., "Maternal Perinatal Risk Factors and Child Abuse" *Child Abuse and Neglect* 9:217-224 (1985); Lewis, E., "Two Hidden Predisposing Factors in Child Abuse," *Child Abuse and Neglect* 3:327-330 (1979); Ney, P., "Relationship Between Abortion and Child Abuse," *Canadian J. Psychiatry* 24:610-620(1979).

30. C. T. Coyle, Ph.D., *Men and Abortion: A Path to Healing* (Belleville, Ontario: Essence Publishing, 1999); Thomas Strahan, "Portraits of Post-Abortive Fathers Devastated by the Abortion Experience," *Assoc. for Interdisciplinary Research in Values and Social Change*, 7(3), Nov/Dec 1994; David C. Reardon, "Forgotten Fathers and Their Unforgettable Children," *The PostAbortion Review* 4(4) Fall 1996.

31. Ibid, 193.

32. Mary Meehan, "Accepting the Unjust," *National Catholic Register*, 18 April 1982.

33. Reardon, *Aborted Women, Silent No More*, 277-278.

CHAPTER FOUR

TESTIMONIES OF RAPE VICTIMS WHO HAD ABORTIONS

When collecting these testimonies, the editors have, of course, honored any requests for anonymity. Names set off in quotes are pseudonyms. All of the names without quotation marks are the women's real names. Many of these women have publicly testified about their experiences in the past; for others, this is the first time they have placed themselves under public scrutiny. The reader will quickly see that most of the women who chose anonymity did so to preserve the privacy of others rather than protect themselves. Whether or not they used their real names, all of these women deserve our respect and admiration for their courage in sharing their stories with us.

"The effects of the abortion are much more far-reaching than the effects of the rape in my life."

—"Patricia Ryan"

Patricia was drugged and raped. When she found herself pregnant, she was urged by Planned Parenthood counselors to have an abortion. Abortion seemed like the best solution at the time, but it turned out to cause more problems than it solved.

I was born and raised in a large Irish-Catholic family. I was one of six children, the oldest daughter, and very mature for my age. When I was only five years old, I was diagnosed with severe asthma, and began a regimen of daily medications.

I had frequent asthma attacks and was severely limited in my physical activities. Even a good, hard laugh could cause me to begin gasping for breath, so when I was fourteen my parents and my doctor decided that as soon as I graduated from high school I would move to Tucson, Arizona to live with my aunt and uncle. It was hoped that the move to a drier climate would allow me to live a more active, healthy life.

I had been a very good student, able to get A's without much trouble or study, and my family and I assumed that I would work my way through the University of Arizona. I was a shy child, and because of my physical limitations I did not participate in sports in school, but I did still have a good amount of friends from a wide cross-section of the student body. I was an editor of the school yearbook, a member of the National Honor Society (from 7th to 12th grade), a student advisor for the psychology department, and graduated among the top students in my class.

One of my greatest interests at that time was a class in criminology that was offered. I decided to study for a degree in psychology, and then join the police force in a brand-new field for crime victims—the Rape Trauma Unit. (How ironic!)

It was with very high expectations that I left Michigan for Arizona, leaving my family and my fiancé, just two weeks past my eighteenth birthday. I lived with my aunt and uncle for three weeks following my arrival in Tucson, then I moved in with three college girls who were renting an apartment close to the store where I had begun working in modeling and cosmetics. Having left a large, close-knit family, plus my boyfriend, I was very lonely and homesick at the time.

While working at the store during the Christmas season of 1974, I met a young woman who invited me to attend a party with her the following weekend. I didn't know her at all, but I was a very trusting, innocent person, and I was excited at the possibility to meet new people and start making friends again.

The night of the party, we went first to an apartment where a party was in progress. When I learned that marijuana was baked into some of the desserts, I asked this young woman if we could leave. Though I had liquor at some of the graduation parties of my friends, I had never tried any drugs—in fact, I was very afraid of them.

She suggested another party that she knew of, at a bar on the outskirts of town. When we arrived, she walked right up to a section of the bar and began to talk with two young men there. I assumed that she was friends with them, and when they offered us some drinks (which were already sitting on the bar), I felt no alarm. I took a sip from one of the glasses and disliked the extremely strong taste of it so I put it back. However, within a few minutes I began to feel extremely light-headed and sleepy.

One of the young men asked if he could drive me home, and

I accepted, since I was becoming scared and disoriented. I was finding it difficult to talk, and the man literally took my arm and guided me toward his car. He took me to an old, ramshackle house near the campus, where I was kept for the night, and he raped me twice.

When I first realized that the man was going to rape me, I was totally terrified, gagging and choking and fighting to breathe. I remember crying through the entire ordeal. I was relieved when he was finally through with me. I prayed throughout the rape, and pictured my family and my boyfriend, and begged God not to let me die. I passed in and out of consciousness, and I don't remember how much time passed, but I came to when he climbed on me again and raped me a second time. Again, I wept through the entire assault, and prayed to survive, my face turned to the wall, just waiting for it to be over.

I must have blacked out again, because the next thing I remember was that it was light in the room and he was up getting dressed. He acted as though there was absolutely nothing wrong with what he had done. I couldn't even bring myself to speak to him. He said that he would drive me to my job, which he did, and that was the last I ever saw of him (except for in my nightmares.) I was so sickened and humiliated by what had happened that I stumbled a mile to my home rather than go in the store for help.

When I finally got to my apartment, all I wanted to do was shower over and over. I cried in my room for days, called in sick to my job, and told no one what had happened to me. Since I had voluntarily gone to the party, and had taken a drink without being forced, I felt that somehow the rape must have been my own fault. The guilt and shame were crushing. I wanted to die. I felt so filthy, so defiled, that I couldn't bring myself to tell even my roommates. I kept my ugly secret to myself, went back to work, and tried to pretend that it had never happened.

Within several weeks of the assault, I realized that I had missed my monthly period, but because of the trauma of the rape, I was sure that my cycle had just been thrown out off by the shock of the attack and that I would return to normal within a month of two. However, when I had missed two additional periods I was forced to accept the possibility that I may have become pregnant from the rape.

I finally confided in my roommates what had happened, and two of them chided me for "making up a big rape story," and told me that "this was a new day and age," that if I just wanted a one-night stand, I didn't have to come up with any excuses for my behavior! My third roommate, Patty, put her arms around me and told me that she would help me any way she could.

I was so grateful for her sympathy and support that when she suggested that I go to Planned Parenthood for a free pregnancy test and counseling, I agreed and went the very next day. Just being there was humiliating. It was so impersonal and cold. I had to wait in a large room with a number of other people while the pregnancy test was being run.

When my number was finally called, I was taken to a small cubicle with two "counselors," who informed me that my test was positive. I was pregnant. I started sobbing, and told them what had happened. When they heard that I had been raped, and that drugs were probably used, they began to question me about how well prepared I was to handle this birth without any support from the father. They asked me if I realized that there could be serious birth defects as a result of the drugs the rapist gave me, and how would I support a child with severe and expensive medical problems. Then, when I felt totally over-whelmed with the hopelessness of my situation, they became very sympathetic and told me that they could make arrange-ments to take care of this problem for me. They said they knew doctors who would terminate the pregnancy, and allow me to go on with my life.

At that point, when I finally felt that there could be an end to the hell that I was living in, I agreed to an abortion. As far as having support during this time, the only options that were pre-sented to me appeared to be: (a) having the baby, and face the tremendous financial burdens of raising a child alone, at eight-een, plus live with the stigma of carrying a rapist's child, and possibly giving birth to a severely handicapped baby, or (b) have a "safe, painless, quick medical procedure" that would allow me to put the whole nightmare behind me. There was really no choice involved.

Two days later, I had a suction and aspiration abortion in a doctor's office. I cried during the procedure, mainly out of fear, and because, contrary to what I had been told, the procedure was excruciatingly painful. It was also nearly as humiliating as the rape itself. The doctor never even looked at me, and the nurses were courteous, but distant and coldly professional.

When I returned home to my apartment, I again went through

a crying jag that lasted several days. At times I felt that I was los-
ing my mind. I suffered from horrifying nightmares of decapi-
tated and dismembered babies calling out to me as they floated,
bleeding, around my dark room. I experienced flashbacks that
were terrifying, and so different from my nightmares. When
something would trigger the flashbacks, I was not just remembering the abortion, *I was back on the table, going through the abortion again!* When I would finally snap out of it, I would be
drenched in sweat and shaking uncontrollably. I began to consider suicide as a means to escape the torment of my own
thoughts and nightmares.

Before long I had to quit my job at the store, because I could-
n't bear the sight of pregnant women or babies in strollers. I
would feel overcome with grief and pain, and I would have to
run to the ladies' room before I blacked out. Also, after the abortion my fears of the rapist returned. Not only did I dream of
dead babies, I also dreamed that the rapist was watching me,
looking in the windows while I slept, waiting around every cor-
ner in the store where I worked.

When I called my parents to ask for the money to fly home to
Michigan again, they were reticent to give me the money and
wanted to know why I needed to come home. Up to this point,
nearly five months after the rape, I still had not told them what
had happened. I was still too ashamed, too crushed. I finally told
my mother that I had been raped, and that I was very afraid that
the rapist would find me again. They did pay my fare to fly
home, but when I arrived and tried to explain what had happened, I was told by my mother not to talk about it again. My
father told me that I was a "slut," a "whore," "that I asked for
it," and that I "had gotten what I deserved."

I was so deeply hurt, that I moved out immediately and got a
flat with a girl I knew. I turned to my boyfriend and to alcohol
for any type of comfort I could get, but my crying, anger and
shame quickly destroyed even that relationship. I felt totally
alone, and wanted only to die.

In my opinion, abortion only compounds the trauma and pain
of rape or incest. I was an innocent victim of a horrible crime. I
was not to blame for what the rapist did to me. But in choosing
to abort, to kill the innocent child growing within me, I lowered
myself to the level of the rapist. I too committed a crime against
a defenseless baby who had done nothing wrong, who was *also*
a victim of the rapist. That child may have been fathered by a

criminal, but I was the mother, and I killed a part of myself when I had the abortion. It only compounded my pain; it didn't solve anything.

I would have to say that I no longer suffer from negative feelings from the rape. That is not to say that it is painless to share my experience, but I have accepted what happened, and I have even seen opportunities to use my experience to help other women who have suffered in similar ways, either through rape or abortion.

I have forgiven the rapist, and I have also forgiven my parents for their lack of compassion and support. I have been able to come to understand the tremendous pain that they experienced upon learning of the assault, and I also understand that they suffered terribly for having made the decision to send me, alone, so far from home, and at such a young and vulnerable age. Our relationship is now close and supportive, even though it is still very painful for them to even mention the rape. It is brought up only *very rarely*.

Given my own experience, I would definitely discourage a woman from having an abortion following rape or incest. While it may appear to be the quickest, easiest solution to a painful, humiliating "problem," it is only a band-aid approach and has terrible ramifications of its own. Instead, I would suggest that she receive counseling from a professional, to help her see that she has been an innocent victim, and that only through seeing the pregnancy through to completion will she really allow herself the chance to heal completely.

I feel that the decision to either keep the baby or give it up for adoption is such an individual one that each case would require careful consideration and prayer. Even though the baby could be a reminder of a very painful event in the life of the mother, I also know of cases where the child of the rapist has been the catalyst to help complete the mother's healing.

In closing, I would like to say that the effects of the abortion are much more far-reaching than the effects of the rape in my life. For a number of years, I have shared my own story to help illustrate the fallacy of abortion as a quick-fix for rape and incest victims. However, at this time, I have had to make some difficult decisions to "phase myself out" of this work. It is not that I am not completely healed, or that I am embarrassed of the events of my past, but that I now have two sons to care for. There is mounting evidence that there is such a thing as "sibling grief," which occurs when prior or subsequent children learn of their mother's abortion. They can very acutely mourn the loss of this brother or sister that they have never known. And they can also experience anxiety from the realization that their mother, who has always embodied stability and security, may actually be someone who has to be feared. Some children live in fear that if they don't perform as expected, "Mommy may get rid of them, too."

I fully credit God with giving me the courage and strength to reach back and face the pain of my past, and my decision to not allow my name to be used in no way negates God's perfect ability to forgive and restore. I am forgiven! That's a fact. And I am living a full and joyful life, with a precious husband and two beautiful children, when fifteen years ago, all I wanted was the peace of death. But my children are now my primary "mission field," and I cannot bear the thought that my past, though forgiven, may undermine the openness and trust that I now share with my sons. I hope that my story may help others.

"Far from helping me deal with the rape and incest, the abortion just covered over the issue ... abortion is not helpful; it only obscures the areas that need healing."
— **Marie Rodier**

Marie was a victim of both incest and rape. Insulted by the police and feeling abandoned by her family, she chose an abortion when she became pregnant after the rape. She found that instead of solving her problems, the abortion merely "put a wall," between her and the issues she needed to face.

Before being raped in 1971, I was living a hippie lifestyle in Berkeley, California. I was 22 years old, single, and living with three people in a co-op apartment. I was living by selling artwork and collecting food stamps. I was part of a women's artistic "consciousness-raising" group and involved in putting together a directory of women artists in the Bay Area. I was 2,000 miles away from my family, and I had no regular boyfriend. There were two men I was involved with sexually, but with no commitment by my choice.

In retrospect, I believe I felt hostility toward men because of my father, who had abused me sexually when I was 13, and who was very critical and controlling. I had been under his influence in college, but since then I had been wildly rebelling for the 20 months since I had graduated in June 1970 from Brown. I spent about half of every week hitchhiking around California to see new places and do landscape painting.

The rape occurred when I was hitchhiking from Berkeley to San Mateo on New Year's Eve 1971. I was making this trip because my father had asked me to pick up some things for him, and since I had no car, I had to hitchhike to get there. I was angry because I no longer wanted him telling me what to do, but I still felt I had to obey him and get this errand out of the way before the year was done; I had already put it off for a month or so. Since I was angry, I felt off-balance and unable to discern the rides I accepted.

The first ride was bad. The second ride picked me up in San Francisco near the city jail. The man was hung over, and he lied to me about where he was going. First he drove to the projects, where he seemed to be looking for an empty room. He didn't tell me anything, but I began to get afraid, and he locked the door on me. Next he drove to a big open field, stopped, and when I refused his advances, he pulled out a knife. We kept wrestling, and I kept trying to get out of the truck. Then he pinned me down on the seat and put the knife to my neck on the right side. I froze in fear. I looked out the window at the blue sky, and decided I wanted to see it some more and to live. I was too afraid to move or to say anything. I let him rape me with the knife at my neck. Then he drove me to the top of some vacant hills and dropped me off. I tried to get the license plate number.

I ran to the nearest house, yelling "help" and crying. A woman took me into her house while we got the police to come. They drove me to the station in downtown San Francisco and on the way, they made sarcastic remarks about how stupid I was to be hitchhiking. That made me feel worse.

At the station I had to wait half-an-hour alone before a staff medical technician examined me. They said they found semen and a red dot on my neck where the knife was, but they didn't think there was enough evidence of rape, especially when I told them I had sex before this even though I wasn't married. After the exam, the police told me that the number of the orange-yellow truck I had given them didn't exist. There was nothing else they could do.

Then the same two officers asked me where I wanted to be

taken, and I gave them the address of a friend who lived in San Francisco. Instead of taking me there, they got me in the car and started making lewd remarks to me as if I was a prostitute, and they dropped me off in front of a hotel where they knew prostitutes hung out. I had no idea where I was, and after asking directions and walking alone for about a mile, I finally arrived at my friend's house. There I took a shower right away, but an hour later I still felt dirty, so I took another shower. I felt defiled, disgusted, and angry. The rape crushed my idealism and trust. I felt betrayed.

I did not contact any assault groups, but I did tell the women in my consciousness-raising group. They mostly supported my feelings of hatred toward men. Someone showed me a few self-defense techniques for the future. They tried to get me to talk about how I felt, but I couldn't.

My family situation really added to the problems. I didn't tell them about it at first because I was angry at my dad for indirectly causing the whole situation. I was afraid to tell him to his face that he had caused it and that I was angry with him. I didn't have any communication with my mom because she had never defended me from my dad. I also had a sinking feeling that I might be pregnant, and I wanted to wait and see.

I found out I was definitely pregnant by getting a test down at the Women's Health Clinic in Berkeley. My immediate feeling was anger; there was never a moment when I thought of the baby as mine. I was as disgusted with the thought of it as I was of the rapist, and I wanted to get rid of it.

I called my mother and told her that I was raped and was pregnant. She asked why they didn't take me in for a D&C, meaning at the police station. I had no idea that was done for rape. She wanted me to keep the baby and offered to raise it herself at home, but I thought that to give my parents a child to raise like they raised us was a fate worse than death, to be beat up and squashed like we were, so I'd rather kill the baby. Also, my dad is quite biased against blacks (the rapist was black) and he would not have treated a biracial child well.

My sister offered to help me raise the baby, but she was living in poverty and drugs with an irresponsible husband and she was younger than me. So I both didn't want to burden her and I was ashamed of myself because so far I had lived by keeping my reputation clean, which she had not, and we'd all judged her. I didn't want to be like her, stuck with a child. I wanted to keep my options open and do things.

My mother wanted to come out to help me with my decision, but since she still had several children at home, my dad wouldn't let her. She feels bad about this even now.

In anger I made the decision alone. When I called my parents, I did so mainly to tell them what had happened knowing it would hurt my dad; it was a form of revenge. In the process of the conversation I realized I had no home to turn to for help or support, so I was alone. I turned to my roommate, who was a feminist and against having children. I didn't really have the support I needed.

My feelings changed from anger into a very withdrawn depression. I had morning sickness and was tired. I felt under pressure internally to abort. I was also influenced by my feminist friends who approved of abortion. However, one feminist I met surprised me by telling me very strongly to consider keeping the baby. I had assumed all feminists approved of abortion; lots of my friends were having abortions for convenience.

I planned from early on to get rid of it. I decided out of anger, wanting to rid myself of the "filth" of this child. Before this I had given no thought to abortion. If it hadn't been that I was raped, I would not have considered abortion, because I did not believe it was moral to abort for convenience. Besides, the state law allowed abortion in cases of rape.

During the abortion I woke up in pain, screaming, "What are you doing to me?" I felt like they had sucked out my guts. The staff was very rude to each other, yelling over the vacuum to hurry up. Afterwards I felt totally empty and stripped of any bit of value in my life. I wanted to go home and start over, so two days after the abortion I went back to Indiana and lived with my sister. I tried to recover the self-worth I'd lost, so I got a job and then went to grad school.

In the years that followed I had no feeling about the political side of the abortion issue. I had no interest in abortion as birth control. To me, all the hoopla about *Roe v. Wade* in 1973 was put on by spoiled liberal rich girls who knew nothing about necessity such as rape. I kept quiet because though I had taken advantage of the California law allowing abortion, I also knew that abortion was not something to treat lightly.

The abortion had negative effects for three years afterwards. Even though I was trying to gain respectability on an outer level, I was also drinking heavily, smoking marijuana, and being promiscuous, even getting involved in three adulterous affairs. It was very depressing.

Another possible effect is that it made relationships with men even more difficult. It took me 15 years to get married. Then when I tried to conceive a child, I discovered I am not able, though my husband and I have not been willing to get all the fertility tests done. We are in our 40s now. This has been a very sad thing to face—that I may have killed my only child. Now I work at a crisis pregnancy center, and I find meaning in trying to help other women avoid the mistakes I made, especially with abortion.

Far from helping me deal with the rape and incest, the abortion just covered over the issue. I started the process of repenting and healing in 1975. I didn't encounter any help in the church until 1989, when I went through the PACE Bible study (a post-abortion Bible study), which has made such a difference. It took me seventeen years to deal with the abortion. Now I am looking at the incest, and I have yet to look at the rape.

I didn't feel much about the rape until I went through the Bible study and saw the connection between the incest and the rape, both of them having to do with my dad. Now as I experience God's forgiveness for my abortion, it has receded as the stressor event. Now I'm dealing with the anger and grief related to the incest, of which I feel the rape is just a continuation and effect. Just a few weeks ago I was I was able to confront my dad in person and tell him about the impact of what he's done to me, my feelings, and about his responsibility in my rape and abortion. That was one step, but I still have a way to go—even though I forgive him—to grieve the loss of trust and childhood and to restore clarity about sexuality in my marriage.

Women who become pregnant as a result of sexual assault should be given intensive emotional care, first for themselves, to deal with the assault first. The assault and the pregnancy should be treated as separate issues, though I know how much the pregnancy becomes the main concern. She needs to know that her child is a separate individual and is not responsible for the circumstances of her conception. She should be helped to acknowledge her maternal instincts (my dad always told me I'd make a terrible mother.)

Abortion is not helpful; it only obscures the areas that need healing by placing a huge wall of guilt between the real issues and the woman's conscience. Abortion puts everyone's attention on the pregnancy instead of on the victim and her needs.

To women who experienced what I did, I'd say be aware of your anger and impatience because they can have worse effects than the rape. Try to get quiet, and be careful of who's pressuring you to do what. Try to hear your conscience and stay in touch with the joy of maternal feelings; don't take your anger out on the baby.

To those who went ahead with the abortion, God knows what went on and He forgives you. What comforts me is the grace of God, the Word of His Truth, and getting good counsel regarding such things as warding off Satan's accusations that I'm not forgiven or that I haven't forgiven others.

I don't feel I made the right decision with the abortion. But it helps me now to have an outlet in a ministry where I volunteer to tell others about my experience and how God has pulled me through it.

"They say abortion is the easy way out, the best thing for everyone, but they are wrong. It has been over 15 years, and I still suffer."

—**"Rebecca Morris"**

Rebecca was raped by a friend and became pregnant. At her mother's urging, she had an abortion, believing that it would solve all her problems. Many years later, she still struggles with the emotional effects of the abortion.

When I was 15 years old, I was raped by a friend of mine. I was a virgin, but I had disobeyed my mother. I was not supposed to have boys in the house after a certain hour.

I had also been drinking that night and smoking marijuana, and as this was the 1970s, my mother was fairly lenient about this. I was to do it at home if I was going to do it.

As I said, this boy was a friend of mine, a very good friend. He had been babysitting for one of our neighbors and I went over to keep him company. We began to drink and get high, and when the parents returned, we went back to my house.

At some point in the evening, we began kissing, and eventually ended up in my bedroom. When things went farther than I wanted, I told him to stop, but he did not. I never thought we would "go all the way," so I didn't get too upset at first, but eventually he got my pants down and was trying to penetrate me. I kept telling him "no" and "stop" but he continued anyway. In fact, I said "no," and "stop" all the way through the act until he was finished. The pain was excruciating, and I hadn't wanted it to happen, but it did. I had tried to push him off me, but that was useless.

He left shortly after he finished and I told no one. No one, that is, until my period didn't come. I went to a nearby clinic six weeks or so later and discovered I was pregnant. I was very scared and confused, and didn't know what to do. I was afraid to tell my mother, but the counselor at the clinic convinced me that I had to.

I told her that night, and we cried together. Then she told me I had to have an abortion. She made all the arrangements, and several weeks later it was all over—or so I thought.

I had been very opposed to abortion under any circumstances, but over the next two-and-a-half years I became pregnant again, through voluntary intercourse. I had my third and final abortion on my 18th birthday.

Shortly after that I became a Christian. I was no longer sexually active and I thought it was all behind me. Certainly when the topic of abortion came up I felt little twinges of guilt, but I tried not to think about it.

I never received any kind of counseling, and finally two years ago, I made an attempt at marriage. I say "an attempt" because it lasted less than a year. I realized shortly after the wedding that I had a rage deep inside me toward men, and it was directed at my husband. I became unable to have sex with him; any attempt at affection felt like intense violation. I realize now that I was re-experiencing all the feelings that surrounded my rape and subsequent pregnancy and abortion.

I have since had a great deal of counseling, and am much better now concerning my feelings toward men and sex, but I have not been able to heal from the abortions.

I am plagued with guilt and regret, and I often think about what I had done to my babies. I frequently calculate in my head how old they would be if I had done the right thing and kept them. It is even more difficult if I see a child that is the same age as mine would be, and think I could have had a son or daughter that age.

For whatever reason, the first abortion bothers me more than the other two, perhaps because I feel it paved the way for the others, or perhaps because each thing that occurred—the rape and the abortion—was against my will.

I am now 31 years old. I think about my children often, and I want an opportunity once more to be a mother. I am at times afraid that my punishment for aborting will be that I am never allowed to conceive another child.

I know the pro-abortionists are wrong. They say abortion is the easy way out, the best thing for everyone, but they are wrong. It has been over 15 years, and I still suffer.

My only comfort is knowing that my babies are in heaven with Jesus. I know He has forgiven me, but I have not yet figured out how to forgive myself.

"The hardest thing of all is trying to forgive myself."
— "Nancy Anders"

Nancy became pregnant as the result of a date rape. She was pressured into an abortion by her family. Feeling guilty and depressed after her abortion, she fell into a life of promiscuity and drug and alcohol abuse.

It was May 1973. I was pregnant from a date rape. I had tried to hide it from my parents but of course they found out. Then the pressure started. "How are you going to go to college with a baby?" "How are you going to support it?" "It is only a blob of blood. It's not a baby yet." Before I had time to think about what *I* wanted, the abortion was over.

The abortion itself was like a living hell. I thought my guts were being pulled out. It was degrading and I was terrified. When it was over, something made me ask the doctor, "Was it a boy or a girl?" He answered, "I can't tell. It's in pieces." The counseling consisted of throwing some birth control pills at me.

It's so hard to put into words how the abortion affected me. Looking back and knowing what I know now, I realize that I was going through almost classic Post-Abortion Syndrome. I became a tramp and slept with anyone and everyone. I engaged in unprotected sex and each month when I wasn't pregnant, I would go into a deep depression. I was rebellious. I wanted my parents to see what I had become. I dropped out of college. I tried suicide. But I didn't have the guts to slit my wrists or blow my brains out. I couldn't get my hands on sleeping pills, so I resorted to over the counter sleep aids and booze.

When that failed, I then tried to make relationships work with men, any man. I was driven by a need to have a child and knew if I was married my parents couldn't do anything about it. Then I married in 1975. While my husband and I are still together, we have had to work extra hard because I married him for all the wrong reasons.

Five months after we were married, my first child was born. I was in heaven. I doted on that baby. In three months, I was pregnant again. But this time we lost our baby at six months. Then the depression that I had conquered came back in full force. I can remember thinking: "I deserve this pain. I killed a baby and now God has taken one from me. I deserve it."

The doctor felt that I had a weak cervix, a common aftereffect of abortion, and that the weight of the baby was too much for it. She just fell out. Four months later I was pregnant again.

It is hard to explain this need to keep having babies, but I did. From 1976, with the birth of my first living child, to 1985, at the birth of my fourth and final living child, I was pregnant a total of eight times. With the birth of my last child the doctor didn't leave me any choice but to quit having children if I wanted to live to see the ones I had grow up.

In trying to deal with the abortion, I had to face what I had done and beg forgiveness from my God. The hardest thing of all is trying to forgive myself. It is a daily struggle to accept the forgiveness I know the Lord has given me. And I will never forget it. Only now I don't want to forget it, because it keeps me from getting complacent. I know if it helps others, I can talk about it. It always makes me cry, but if it saves just one mom and baby the pain, it's worth it.

I joined our local Right to Life and a crisis pregnancy center. I have also had to forgive my parents. I can still remember when I walked into my mom's house and threw down a picture of an aborted fetus and snarled, "See what you made me do?" She has since become pro-life herself and has told me how sorry she is. I still have to fight against my anger at my dad, because he still won't admit the abortion was wrong, at least for me.

Do all these things help? That's a hard one. Sometimes it does and sometimes the depression is too strong and time has to pass. Not a day goes by that the abortion doesn't cross my mind. It is a constant struggle trying to overcome my guilt and depression, even knowing I have been forgiven. I dread the day when I have to come to face to face with my little child and explain to her why mamma took her life. But I also think I am a softer, more caring person than I might have been. If not for the abortion, I might have turned out "pro-choice."

"Abortion does not help or solve a problem—it only compounds and creates another trauma for the already grieving victim by taking away the one thing that can bring joy."
—Helene Evans

Helene was raped while on a date during her freshman year of college. When she found out she was pregnant, she went to a "counselor" for help, only to be told that abortion was her only option. Too ashamed to face her parents, she reluctantly went ahead with the procedure. Today she says that although she no longer suffers from the rape, she still struggles with the effects of the abortion on a daily basis.

I grew up in a church-going family, but not a Christ-centered home. I was a good kid; I feared my father and I did everything I could not to upset him. I had my days when I was very ornery, and I liked to see how far I could push the limits, but when it came down to the line, "no" meant no, and I listened. In high school I excelled in sports and academics. I had good friends—there were plenty of opportunities to get into trouble, but there was a group of us who liked to just hang out and we really had no problems staying away from the wrong influences. We had fun just being who we were.

I had only dated very briefly in high school; they were very good innocent experiences. I believe it was because I had a wonderful Sunday School teacher. She talked with us about the blessings of how God intended sex for marriage and the joy of waiting for marriage. Her words penetrated my heart and I knew it was the right thing to do. Overall I breezed through high school, was accepted into a college and was very excited about my future.

My sexual assault was what has been titled date or acquaintance rape. My freshman year of college I was dating a young man who I had met that previous summer. We had talked about what we believed in and he knew my convictions about saving sex for my husband. Yet after a few months of dating he became impatient with waiting and forced himself on me against my protest. After the assault I blamed myself for letting it happen; I felt it was my fault and that I could have somehow avoided it. I did not realize until much later that it was a rape. I was scared of him; therefore, I did not tell anyone what had happened.

Two months later I became sick with the flu, only this flu did not go away. It was in the bathroom stall of our local mall that I first learned of my pregnancy. A fear gripped me like none I had ever known. My head was spinning, my heart was pounding, and I was alone and terrified. Where could I go? Who could I tell? My parents would kill me. How could I explain how it happened? It was already August and I would be returning to college in only a few weeks. I had to find help quickly.

Not knowing where to go for help, I went to the phone book, found the first place that offered pregnancy testing and counseling and made an appointment. I was looking for someone who could give me direction and guidance. Unfortunately the only option that was offered by the counselor was abortion. Her solution was abortion now or later—later would, according to her, require hospitalization.

I panicked when I heard this. My parents would find out if I waited. I couldn't face that so I chose what I thought was my only option. Extremely distressed, tears streaming down my face, stifling the sobs that were now coming, I signed the papers. A young girl in a crisis situation, obviously distressed . . . a box of Kleenex was the extent of the counsel I received. Alone, in a strange place, still in shock from finding out I had conceived, I made a decision that will be with me for the rest of my life.

Prior to my pregnancy I did not agree with abortion, but I never thought I would have to make that decision. I did not want an abortion, but I felt I had no other choice.

After the abortion, I wanted to die. How could I live when I had just ended the life of my child? The negative feelings resulting from the rape were not eliminated by the abortion. Nothing was solved; instead, the grief was now doubled. I became severely depressed and suicidal. The pain was so intense that I would cut myself. Somehow this helped release all that was locked inside that I could not express.

I was back at college, halfway into the first semester of my sophomore year. I had been an excellent student the year before, and now I was beginning to fail my classes. My professors were concerned, but did not know what to do. My parents still had no idea [what had happened.] Finally a concerned friend, who saw the changes taking place and recognized my need for help, confronted me. She too had been raped and could identify with my pain. She took me to a counselor, and thus began the long process of healing.

I no longer have negative feelings about the rape. Yes, I wish it did not happen, but it is in the past and God has healed that, and I have moved on. It is the abortion that I still struggle with on a daily basis. It is difficult for me, when I see a child, not to wonder what mine would have looked like. When I start to dream about how beautiful she would be, I remember the reason why she is not here. It is a daily battle of taking my sin, my guilt, my shame and laying it down at the cross where it was paid for and letting my Savior wash it all away, and then walking away whole and restored.

In my opinion an abortion is never, in any circumstances, a good solution to rape or incest or any crisis pregnancy. An abortion only adds to and compounds the trauma that has already occurred. A woman, who has already been violated once, does not benefit from the violent loss of her innocent child. God gave every woman a special ability to bond with a child even before it is born. Even though she may not confess it with her mouth, I believe deep down inside a woman knows this is a baby and not just a bundle of cells. So when it is ripped away by an abortion, a bond is broken and grief will occur.

I feel those who support abortion in cases of rape and incest do not know what they are talking about. What they may think is an act of mercy, is no mercy at all. Abortion does not help or solve a problem—it only compounds and creates another trauma for the already grieving victim by taking away the one thing that can bring joy.

I believe that it is actually healing for a woman who has suffered a traumatic pregnancy to see the life she can bring into this world and to experience the joy that comes with that new life. People need to remember that there is a God who can take what Satan meant for evil and turn it into a beautiful, wonderful thing.

To those women who are dealing with a pregnancy as a result of a rape or incest: you are not alone. We have a God who knows us more intimately than any person ever could. He knows our deepest needs and is longing for you to know Him. He is the only one who can heal those deep wounds, and I believe rape, incest and abortion cause deep wounds to our souls. True healing can only come from the Ultimate Counselor Himself. If we allow Jesus Christ to be a part of our healing process we can be whole again.

"I tried for years to drown the guilt and pain I felt in drugs and alcohol. But it got to the point where there wasn't enough alcohol, weren't enough drugs, weren't enough cigarettes to dull the pain."

—Debby Enstad

Debby was raped while living as a college student in Mexico. When she discovered she was pregnant, she had an abortion. For the next two decades she experienced drug and alcohol abuse, suicide attempts, a failed marriage, and another abortion. Now she wants to tell other women that abortion is not a "quick, easy fix," but a mistake that can lead to a lifetime of suffering.

I was in college when I came home to my apartment one evening and found that my roommates were having a party. I wanted to leave and get something to eat, but my friends had loaned my car to someone else. I was going to call a taxi when a couple of men there said they would give me and my two friends a ride. We left my friend Nancy off first, and then stopped for tacos at an outdoor stand.

When we stopped for gas later, I thought I saw that one of them had a handgun, but I thought it couldn't be, so I just dismissed it. We drove back toward my apartment. My friend Richard and I were in back, and as I was thanking the others for the ride, the driver suddenly swung his arm back, put a gun to Richard's forehead, and said, "get out." I put my hand on the driver's arm, to see what we were dealing with. I could feel he was ready to shoot, and I knew it would kill Richard. So I told him to get out, that I would be all right.

Richard told them, "You're crazy," and then I saw the fire from the gun. Richard crumpled to the ground, and I thought he was dead. I started screaming. They said they'd killed Richard and they would kill me.

I believe in God, and I began to pray; I knew my life was on the line.

One of them started raping me with a gun to my head, while the other drove off. They took me somewhere—to this day I don't know where—and more people said they wanted to rape me. For the next twelve hours it went on. Seven people raped me.

The only way I survived that long night was through prayer. I thought, "You don't really have me. You just have a body, a rag doll. You don't have my heart, my soul, my mind, my desires. You don't have *me*." I believe I made it through what I did because of prayer.

After twelve hours, something happened so they just couldn't kill me, couldn't hurt me. They carried me back to the car. They were even gentle with me. I knew it was the hand of God. He made it so that in their hearts they couldn't kill me.

The driver who shot Richard took me back to my apartment. He told me, "I killed your friend, and I want you, too. I am coming back for you." I wanted him to come back, too, because I wanted to kill *him*.

I tried to find Richard. The woman across the street told me Richard was in a hospital, and I went from one place to another until I finally found him. The newspaper said he was dead and that I was the only witness alive. They said that a gang was responsible and that my life was in jeopardy. The police said I had to go into hiding.

I went to another large city some distance away. I couldn't go home. I couldn't function, couldn't talk. When I found out I was pregnant I wrote to a girlfriend who is a registered nurse, and she came to help me. She decided I should have an abortion, and took me to San Diego where I talked with Planned Parenthood. They set up the abortion. They said it wouldn't hurt me, doesn't hurt the baby and that I'd feel better afterwards.

I had only $50, so that's what they charged me. I remember lying there in the doctor's office. No nurse, no one else around. I remember horrendous pain, and I was thinking, "I'm going to die." I know I felt I needed to die because I was killing my baby. "Let me die," I prayed.

I didn't die, and I was disappointed. I bled for three days, and went to see friends in Sacramento. I thought again I was dying, bleeding to death, and called my mom in Washington, only to say goodbye, and that I loved her. After I hung up the phone, I went unconscious.

My friends found me and took me to the emergency room. They did surgery, and when I came to, I was disappointed again—I was still alive. Again I quit talking, would hide from people. I wanted to die so bad, wanted to get up and cut my wrists, and then the hurting could stop.

My pain was not because of the rape, or the shooting, but because of the abortion. I couldn't live with what I had done. I wanted to die, but I felt that if I took my life, I really would not get to heaven. So I tried to trick God.

I took a whole handful of pills—uppers, downers, all kinds. And I swallowed them and said, "Lord, you know it's a possibility I may not wake up tomorrow. But you know if I don't, it was an accident."

Again, I didn't die. I went home, and finally faced my mother. "I told her about the rape and everything, and she said, "Don't tell anybody. They'll judge you."

I camped out for a time, living in my Volkswagen bus, mostly in the mountains of Lake Tahoe. I had stopped talking and I had very little money. I got my food from the back of grocery stores. I learned that they threw away expired foods like yogurt, and I would eat that.

Then one day my best friend got mad at me, shook me and said, "I know you. I know you can talk." I began to realize that the only way I could make sense out of everything I had been through was by helping someone else.

I went back to college, where I got my bachelor's degree in nursing and another bachelor's degree in human services. Just before I finished school, I got pregnant again and had another abortion. I tried for years to drown the guilt and pain I felt in drugs and alcohol. But it got to the point where there wasn't enough alcohol, weren't enough drugs, weren't enough cigarettes to dull the pain.

The more mistakes I made the deeper I got, the more worthless I felt. I was always trying to fix my life, always looking for cures. I was always trying to find love—the only way I felt validated was if someone wanted me.

I got married and had two children, but I continued to drink. I couldn't forgive myself for the abortions. My husband and I eventually divorced, but then I found out I was pregnant again. I felt completely alone. I felt the shame. Everyone in town quit talking to me. I was working as a psychiatric nurse, and cried while driving back and forth to work every day. There are so many liberals and humanists who say that it's all right to be pregnant, divorced and unmarried with kids, but I knew it wasn't.

People, including my mother, told me, "You are alone,

divorced, no family." They said, "Who will be there in the labor room, afterwards? You are alone." But I said I wouldn't have another abortion. Rape is wrong, and abortion didn't make it right. It made it worse. That's the part I couldn't live with all these years.

This time, I said, I've done something wrong, but I'm not going to do something wrong on top of it— kill a baby. This time I'm going to do the right thing.

My daughter is a total blessing. I didn't deserve her, but I thank God for her and for my other children. I thought, after my abortions, how could God trust me with another baby? And now my children are my greatest blessings.

I said, "I'm sorry, Lord," and turned my life over to Him. People were wrong when they said no one would be there for me. God was there. He was with me during my pregnancy, my labor, and afterwards.

Some people think we Christians are self-righteous, intolerant, non-compassionate, biased about abortions, because they say we don't care about the woman. But that's why I *do* care about abortion. I *do* care about the woman—because I am that woman.

With abortion your thinking gets twisted—here I was coming from an upright background and I find myself killing my baby. Abortion opens the door to the enemy. Satan gets a foothold in your life—a terrible foothold grounded in murder.

So many times women say they support legal abortion because if their daughters ever became pregnant, they would want abortion to be available for them. I want to tell those moms, "Abortion will not help your daughters. It will only make their problems worse."

People think that abortion is a quick, easy fix. It doesn't help. With pregnancy, I only suffered for a short time during the pregnancy itself. When my children were born they were great blessings and the suffering was gone. With abortion you will suffer for the rest of your life.

CHAPTER FIVE

TESTIMONIES OF RAPE VICTIMS WHO GAVE BIRTH TO THEIR CHILDREN

"Once the baby continued to kick and move, I began to have different feelings toward the child. I began to realize that this little life inside me was struggling too. Somehow, my heart changed."

—Kathleen DeZeeuw

Kathleen was brutally raped. It was six months before she was able to confront the fact that she was pregnant. At first she wanted an abortion, but then decided to place the child for adoption. At the last minute, her love was so great she insisted that she would raise him herself. It has not always been easy for Kathleen and her son Patrick, but she has no doubt that he has been her greatest blessing.

I am Kathleen DeZeeuw. I am married and have three sons (two of whom are married) and one darling granddaughter. In 1963, I was the victim of sexual assault—namely rape.

My life prior to the sexual assault was a normal young Midwest girl's life. I was the sixth child in a family of eight children. I was raised in a "Christian" home. My parents were very strict with us, not ever allowing us to date or be friends with anyone who was not of our particular church. My main interest as a young girl was music. I loved playing the piano and, as a result, found "fixing" them, and ultimately tuning them, a main love.

I was shy and introverted, mainly because from the time I was in eighth grade I was tall and thin. This affected many of my relationships with others around me. I rarely ever dated because we were very restricted as to whom we were allowed to be with. But, nevertheless, I had all the dreams of one day "falling in love" with my knight in shining armor, marrying, and living in a house with the proverbial white picket fence. This dream was short-lived, for within days of my sixteenth birthday my life

74

would be forever changed.

One night a girlfriend and I skipped out on a church meeting and went to a coffee house where many of the town's young people met. Here I accepted a movie invitation with a guy whom I really didn't know. Once at the drive-in movie I realized he had been drinking heavily, and, in fact, carried a lot of liquor with him in the car. It was also here that I found out he had just recently been released from prison. His liquor-induced state was a frightening experience for me, but it wasn't until I asked him to take me back to my own car that I realized what danger I was really in. Instead of returning me, he took me out to a remote area.

After I had my head bashed against a window repeatedly, was raped, and then thrown from the car, I picked myself up and went home. I was left a shattered, frightened person. I felt dead inside. Everything within me was shattered and dirty. He had stolen from me something I could never get back.

What was worse was that my disobedience had led to the rape. Consequently, I blamed myself. Since I wasn't "dragged off the street" I figured it wasn't a "real" rape. It must have been all my fault! So I hid my guilt and shame.

As a result of my own fear and shame at having defied my parents' rules, I didn't report the rape. I just went home and became even more introverted. I didn't tell a single person what had happened to me. In fact, no one knew I was pregnant until I was about six and a half months along.

I had carefully concealed the shame and horror of this assault, as well as the baby that had been conceived by it, for over half a year. I lived in constant fear because this guy, just released from prison, warned me what he could do to me. For a 16-year-old girl, this was warning enough. I was also afraid of how my father might react to my being in a place forbidden to me. Between these two fears, I was in constant terror.

But after six and a half months, the secret could no longer be hidden. My family's reactions were very diverse. My mother wanted to kill herself. My father cried. My brothers and sisters acted as if I had a disease. Many in the community treated me as though I were a whore. Because I wouldn't talk about it, many rumors started about me and everyone had his own interpretation of what must have "really" happened. In the end, I was sent to a home for unwed mothers, in a state a thousand miles away.

My family's rejection of me made me even more reclusive.

This began a course of hatred and bitterness on my part. I didn't trust anyone. It seemed as though no one cared about what had really happened.

During the first six months after the assault, I lived with yet another fear: that was the terrible fear of being pregnant with this person's child. I lived in a state of denial at first and then, when my periods didn't come, I began a path of self-destruction and destruction of the child that was growing inside of me.

I knew, when I was being raped, that I'd become pregnant. I remember screaming this over and over again. This only served as a terrifying source of hideous laughter from the guy who was raping me. This very laughter would haunt me in the years to come.

As a result of all the fear, I tried on my own to abort this man's child. I swallowed bottles of aspirin and a bottle of ant poison; I jumped off haystacks and out of the top part of a hay barn—all to no avail. It wasn't until I felt the life inside me begin to kick that I fully realized that my worst nightmare was indeed true: I was really pregnant! Words can never truly describe the horror this brought me.

However, once the baby continued to kick and move, I began to have different feelings toward the child. I began to realize that this little life inside me was struggling too. Somehow, my heart changed. I was no longer thinking of the baby as the "rapist's." Maternal bonding began in this 16-year-old girl. To this day that, too, is hard to describe.

I no longer wanted to abort this child. I was the only one who had ever considered it. There was, however, a lot of emphasis on adoption. In fact, that was the reason that I was sent to a home for unwed mothers. My parents sent me there after members of our church and the community encouraged them in this direction.

When I was sent to the home in Michigan, an even stronger bond developed between me and the child. I now thought of this baby as "my baby." My baby was all that I had. I felt abandoned by everyone. I had only the life inside me to talk to. It was just us two.

I wasn't one to make friends with others easily, especially after being abandoned, as it were, by my family and friends. My two girl friends had also turned their backs on me so I had little trust in anyone.

When the time of the birth arrived, I spent 27 hours in labor, once again alone. When Patrick was born, he nearly lost his life by strangulation, as the umbilical cord was wrapped many times around his neck. I remember them frantically rushing him from the delivery room.

This was another difficult thing to deal with. I'd grown to love this child and even though I'd tried to abort him, now he was a part of me and I didn't want him to die. I just wanted to see him, to hold him. However, he was temporarily taken away. I thought I would never get to see or hold him.

The following ten days were days of a different kind of torment. This baby, whom I'd grown to care for, was now off-limits. I could only view him from a distance of about 20 feet and only through a very small window. I can't begin to explain the very strong maternal feelings I had for my son. This little one had come from my womb. He'd fought hard to get this far. We'd been through a lot together. We were *both* victims of this assault.

For ten long days, I lived separated from everyone I loved: my family, my friends, and now the little one I'd carried for nine long months.

My parents drove to Michigan to bring me back home. When they arrived, we met with the case worker. There was a family waiting for me to relinquish my rights to what would then have been their son. After that meeting I asked my parents if they would go with me to look at the baby through the window. My father didn't want to see him or have anything to do with "this child." This caused me to feel even more rejected and confused. This ended with my parents leaving for their motel and my going back to my lonely room.

The night before I was to sign my baby away, I couldn't sleep well and, because I had been raised in a home where prayer was important, I asked God to show me what to do. My father also struggled with God that night and later told me he'd walked the floor all night, asking God to show him what he and my mother were to do about this baby, their first grandson.

The Creator of Life heard my prayer and in two distinct dreams that night showed me I was to keep and raise my son. My father also felt as though we, as a family, were to face this together.

My reception at home, however, was not very welcomed by certain other family members. Now I had brought this "bastard" child home. There were many hard times ahead.

This decision was not going to be an easy one. Up until the

decision to keep Patrick had been made, I still wasn't allowed to see or hold him. When my parents told the case worker that we were going to keep Patrick, only then was I allowed to hold him.

The first time I held him, I was instantly reminded of his conception. This tiny baby was an identical replica of his father. I can still remember the revulsion I felt at first. This was something I now had to again face on a daily basis. I'll not tell you it was never a problem for me, for it was. There were many times as my child was growing up that I had terrible feelings of hatred toward him. Often I was reminded through a look on his face. The laughter of my little boy often reminded me of the hideous laughter of this guy as he had raped me.

I always had to consciously remember that it was not Patrick's fault. I failed at this many times and took my hatred out on an innocent child. I had many emotional problems that had to be worked through. This took *time*. This, I found out in retrospect, is one of the most important gifts a person has.

I'm not proud of the fact that I had tried to abort my child. I'm sorry to say that at the time, had abortions been readily available as they are today, I'm afraid my son would not be living. I can only thank God that wasn't an available option for me, because had it been, just when I was most vulnerable, I might have ended the life of my son. Nearly every time I see my son's radiant smile and see his love of life, I'm reminded of the fact that I tried to still that life.

As I stated before, *time* is of great importance. Had I been successful in snuffing out the life of Patrick, I would have never had the opportunity to see this vastly important truth.

I can honestly say my heart grieves for the woman who is so desperate that she feels that abortion is her only option. She too is at one of the most vulnerable times of her life. However, if she is given the *time* and is supported in her *self-sacrifice*, she too will be able to one day look back and be glad that she saved this precious life.

Time and self-sacrifice. I'm not implying that everyone should keep and raise their baby. I, for one, know how very difficult that can be. Yet there are homes ready and waiting for children—empty arms needing to be filled with the gift of life. So time and sacrifice could mean only nine months out of one's life. Even this may be a burden, but at least in this way she would not incur the additional pain of subjecting herself to yet another violent act.

Women who have gone through the trauma of rape or incest need to be counseled, cared for, and listened to. If they conceived, they need to be encouraged to work through their anger and bitterness. I believe that to encourage a woman to have an abortion is to add even more violence to her life. The fact that she is still alive should give her an added reason to cherish the innocent life growing inside her as well. Two wrongs will never make a right.

I personally believe that for her child's sake, she should strongly consider adoption. That may sound strange coming from me, but I know the emotional problems that can result from being daily reminded of the assault. In many cases it may be truly better for the child that he or she not be subjected to this added turmoil.

I am not sorry, nor ever will be, that I kept and raised my son. The life I tried to snuff out was the very tool that was used to bring me to a place where I could forgive those involved in what happened to me. God truly did work it out.

Still, I regret the things I put my son through because of my unforgiveness toward the man who raped me. It took me many years to come to grips with my own problem, which meant I had to quit blaming him for all my emotional problems. I had many years of analysis to try and overcome my deep-seated hatred and bitterness. I lived much of this time in a drug and alcoholic stupor, because I had buried the anger I had toward everyone who I thought had let me down.

It was Patrick, my son, conceived in rape—whose life I had tried to snuff out—who taught me how to forgive. He was willing to forgive not only his biological father, but also me (for physically and verbally abusing him as a child). He kept telling me, "Mom, you need to forgive." Finally I listened to his most sound advice. It was then that I was able to go on with life and to forgive as I had been forgiven. Patrick was God's tool to help me find peace.

My son is truly an example of God's great love and grace. He is not a "misfit" nor has he, in any way, gone the way of his biological father. His life, as everyone's, is truly unique and special. I'm so very blessed by and proud of my son.

To me, it is an affront every time I hear all the rhetoric from the pro-abortionists. I, having lived through a rape, and also having raised a child "conceived in rape," feel personally assaulted and insulted every time I hear that abortion should be legal because of rape and incest. I feel that we're being used to further the abortion issue, even though we've not been asked to tell our side of the story.

As I stated before, a woman is most vulnerable at a time such as this, and doesn't need to be pounced on by yet another act of violence. She needs someone to truly listen to her, care for her, and give her *time* to heal.

I am now the assistant director of a crisis pregnancy center. In that role, I've had many opportunities to counsel victims of rape and incest. I tell them what I've just told you—that given time, care and concern, and love, they too can and do recover. But for them to go through yet another act of violence will never undo the violence that was done to them.

"I thank God for the strength He gave me to go through the bad times and for all of the joy in the good times. I will never regret that I chose to give life to my daughter."
—**Mary Murray**

Mary was raped by a soldier while stationed with her army husband in Germany. After her daughter was born, her husband left rather than accept the child as a part of their family. However, another man came into her life who loved and accepted all her children. Today, Mary is happy and thankful that she made the decision to raise her child.

In the fall of 1979 I was living as the wife of an army serviceman stationed in Germany. I was 24 years old and the mother of three daughters.

While my husband was away on CQ duty our home was broken into by another soldier who we later found out was in my husband's same unit. He broke into our home through a dining room window. I was asleep on the sofa with our youngest daughter who was ill and fussy, while my other two daughters were asleep in their room. I was beaten and assaulted at knife point, and my baby's life was threatened if I didn't cooperate.

I did not seek immediate attention medically or from the police. I felt a lot of fear that the rapist would return, because I might be able to identify him since he hadn't been disguised. Instead, I waited for my husband to return the next day, and he reported it. I was taken to the base clinic and later transferred to another hospital at a nearby base. The doctor was very unfriendly and made me feel like "I'd asked for it" in some way, and the police were pretty much the same. I felt dirty, used, and abused. For weeks afterwards I was depressed and angry.

There were no support groups to help me. I went to the only army counselor and his advice was for me to take a two week vacation, during which time I'd forget it ever happened. No one, including me, knew what to say or do. My parents and family were thousands of miles away in the U.S. I needed someone who'd "been there" to talk to, but there was no one.

The CID investigator assigned to the case was wonderful. He was very quiet and calm and gathered enough evidence for an airtight case. However, the company commander had the man transferred out of the country before he could be prosecuted. He is still out there somewhere!

After the rape, I missed two cycles, but thought it was due to stress. I couldn't accept the possibility that I might be pregnant. After I missed my third cycle, I went to the doctor and was hospitalized with a severe cervical infection. They talked about a hysterectomy. At that time I found out I was pregnant.

I was at first shocked, and then scared of how my husband would react. He'd had a vasectomy, so there was no doubt of when I'd conceived. The logical part of me I knew I'd have and keep the baby, but the emotional part of me didn't know how I was going to do it. I've never believed in abortion and I couldn't give up a child I'd carried to term. I had no idea how to tell my husband and family. I knew they would not agree with me.

Abortion was very strongly encouraged by the military medical personnel, as well as by my husband and family. My husband said, "Abortion *now*," while I was still in the hospital. He called my parents, who agreed with him. I was told I was emotionally unable to make the decision, so my husband would make it for me. I checked myself out of the hospital to escape a forced abortion. I could not rationalize how the violent act committed against me gave me the right to commit a violent act against an innocent child; a child that was part of me.

In the early months of the pregnancy, I was anxious. I did not know how to feel about the baby; it was different than with my other girls. But as I began to feel life, I fell in love with my baby. I had forgotten that she was *my* child too. Once I realized that, I began to feel excited about the birth, although I did worry about "bad genes," how the baby would look (the rapist was black, I was white), what people would say, etc.

Once everyone knew how I felt about abortion, the push for adoption began. Most of the pressure came from my husband and family. I bet I was told a million times that I couldn't raise a "mixed" child with my blond-haired, blue-eyed daughters, because everyone would "know" she was not my husband's.

I never really got over the anger that my attacker got off when we had an airtight case. He never had to pay for what he did, and I had to live with it forever. But I did learn not to associate my feelings about the attack with my feelings about the pregnancy. She did not ask to be conceived.

When my daughter was born, my decision to keep her cost me my marriage. When she was six weeks old my husband told me to make a choice—him or the baby. I chose my child and we separated and eventually divorced. I have custody of all four girls.

On the plus side, my daughter's birth brought me the support of a family friend who fell in love with her at first sight, and gave her the attention she wasn't getting from my husband.

Do I regret the decision to have and keep my child? NO. I heard stories of how "I'd look at her/him and see the rapist," or "take my anger at the rapist out on him/her." Maybe those things do happen for some women, but not to me. I look at my daughter and see the gentle, beautiful spirit God gave her.

When people meet my children, they are always drawn to her. I cannot explain the reason for this, but it happens all the time. It is not because she looks "different" from my other three "white" children—I am remarried and my husband is a beautiful black Christian man who has legally adopted her. He has raised her since she was three-and-a-half months old, but waited until she was five years old to adopt her so that she would understand how special she is to him.

I worried about the "genetic" scares people tell you about: how the child could inherit the father's violent behaviors, etc. But I believe God has truly blessed my daughter's birth with life. Her spirit is one of quiet gentleness. She is slow to anger. She loves spending her time at nursing homes, visiting her many "adopted grandparents" there. She is willing to help anyone in any way she can. At ten years old she has learned more about giving love than many adults I know.

My greatest concern was how I would tell her about her conception. How do you tell a child who wants to know about her "real" dad, that he was a rapist? This is where being a Christian really makes a difference.

I became involved with "Texas Rescue," a part of the national group of Operation Rescue. Through my experiences as a rescuer, my children learned all the true facts of abortion. When word got out through the adults in Texas Rescue about my story, I was asked to do a NBC interview. The catch was that they also wanted to interview my daughter, and she had not yet been told about her conception.

I knew the importance of letting people know that children of rape are happy, beautiful, normal children, so I wanted to do the interview, yet I didn't know if my daughter was ready to handle the "truth." I sought out advice from those whom I knew walked closely with the Lord at my church and my rescue friends. In the end my husband and I decided we would tell her and let her make the decision on the interview. We then prayed for God's timing in telling her.

Two days later, totally unexpected, my daughter asked me why she was adopted, and what happened to her "real" dad. It looked like God's timing! I was able to spend quite a while alone with her and explain to her what I felt she could understand about her conception, birth, adoption, and even the difficult times when I was being pressured to abort her.

I was truly amazed at the way she listened and responded. Her greatest response to me was that she wanted to do the interview so that she could tell others that even if they don't have a "good daddy" to begin with, God can give them a "good daddy" like he gave to her when she was adopted. That every child is His child and He will take care of us, no matter how we began. Such wisdom from a 10-year-old child! Her dad and I are very proud of her. In no way do I regret the decision to give her life and raise her.

Yes, I regret my divorce and the separation of my other children from their father. But God saw to it that a man of God entered my life at the time I needed Him to and all five of our children are being raised by a wonderful "daddy."

My children and I feel very lucky. I know there are other women raising their children alone, and some of those children were conceived like my daughter was. I pray that each of them knows what a precious gift these children are to our God, and how lucky we are to have the privilege of raising them for Him.

These past ten years have not always been easy. I still relive the night of my rape if I happen to see a TV show on the subject.

I have to deal with a bitter, angry ex-husband who has since abused my older children during his visitations, resulting in our needing to move to another state. After that the courts stopped his visits, forcing him into counseling.

It was six years before my father would even speak to me again because I was divorced. "Friends" (those I thought were friends) won't even speak to me because of my "mixed" children and black husband. But through it all, I see my daughter. I see her smile. I see her loving nature. I see her walk with our Lord.

I thank God for the strength He gave me to go through the bad times and for all of the joy in the good times. I will never regret that I chose to give life to my daughter. I pray some day that abortion will no longer be a "choice," and that the world will come to know how precious every gift of life is to our Maker.

"I think that rape victims with pregnancies are discriminated against because people seem to think you're nuts to have a baby by a man who raped you. We are looked upon as being liars, or stupid."

—Sharon "Bailey"

At the age of 15, Sharon was raped by an acquaintance. A quick marriage to another man made it relatively easy for her to decide to keep her baby. But the marriage was rocky, perhaps due in part to her husband's resentment toward her daughter. Looking back, Sharon feels her daughter may have had a more normal life if she had been placed for adoption. Sharon's daughter describes her views later in this book under the name "Beth Bailey."

I was raised in a Christian home. My parents were active in the church. I was somewhat rebellious. I knew that what the church taught was true, but I didn't want to live a Christian life and resented being "forced" to go to church.

Before I was raped, I didn't have an interest in much of anything but boys. I went to church every Sunday morning and night and every Wednesday night. I was a fairly typical 15-year-old girl. I spent most of my time with my two best friends and when I wasn't with them I was on the phone.

Most of my friends considered me to be sweet and innocent.

They did drugs, smoked, drank, and were sexually active. They seemed to respect, even admire, me because I didn't do these things. No one ever ridiculed me because I didn't. I used to say that if they wanted to be sexually active I had no problem with it, but I was going to be a virgin when I got married, even if I was the last one.

I was 15 when I was raped. It was a July afternoon. A friend of mine called and asked me to come over and meet an out-of-town friend. I had faced problems with Mike before, but he was married now with a baby on the way, so I thought he'd be okay. He lived a few houses down the street from me so I walked down.

After I was there a little while Mike asked me to go upstairs with him because he wanted to talk to me about his friend. When I hesitated, he said sarcastically, "Don't worry, I'm not going to rape you." This was a guy I wanted approval from. He was 18, good-looking, charming, popular, and on the football team. So regardless of the pit in my stomach I followed him up stairs.

As soon as we got upstairs, he started to undress me. I thought I could talk him out of it, but he wasn't hearing anything I said. When I realized that he was going to succeed at what he had planned, I couldn't believe it. I kept asking him to not do this. But he did.

As soon as he realized that I was a virgin, he stopped. All I could do was cry. He put his arms around me and he kept telling me how sorry he was. I didn't know if he was really sorry or if he was just scared.

As I walked home, I tried to decide what I was going to do, if anything. I was scared. I don't know why but I knew that he wouldn't bother me anymore. Nevertheless, I was scared. I thought that if I told my mother she would blame me, because she really liked him. But if I didn't tell anyone, I wouldn't have to talk about it. And I figured that if I got married in three years, my future husband probably couldn't tell that I wasn't a virgin. Within minutes I decided that it never happened.

This denial, or blocking out of the reality of it all, worked for a short period of time. A few days, maybe. I had it so far back in my mind that I could even see Mike on the street and not think about it. As a result, I didn't have much feeling about it, except for maybe feeling stupid.

After I realized I might be pregnant, I told my two best

friends. They were in shock. They were more upset than I was. Mary's reaction was, "I can't believe this happened to you." Karen's was, "I'm gonna kill him!"

Shortly after I was raped (about two weeks) I started seeing a guy named Joe. I wasn't allowed to date yet but he came to my house every night. After I realized I might be pregnant, I told him what had happened. He asked me to marry him, if I was pregnant, and that we'd tell everyone that the baby was his. As it turned out I did marry him. He was 20. I was 15.

Joe made arrangements with Birthright for me to have a pregnancy test. After they did the test, the counselor came in the room and shut the door. I knew then what she was going to say. We didn't tell her what really happened. She thought we were just another young couple with an unexpected baby. As she talked to Joe, I stared into space. I couldn't believe it! Not me! My parents will kill me!

My mind was awhirl. At first, as I talked to Joe about us getting married, I began to feel it was our baby. My surface feelings were happiness. I was getting married and we were going to have a baby.

My mother wanted to send me to a Christian home for unwed mothers and have the baby put up for adoption. I had already decided to keep it. She insisted for months that I could never handle having a baby. Finally, my mother reluctantly agreed to let us get married and keep the baby.

As for abortion, I didn't even consider it. I felt very strongly about abortion. On most topics I was wishy-washy, but I was solid on my opposition to abortion. I felt that a baby is a baby, totally innocent, no matter how they are conceived. Besides, how could I kill my own baby?

I was three months pregnant when we got married. Joe was very supportive during my pregnancy. I felt he would always take care of me and the baby.

When I was four months pregnant I started bleeding. I cried because I thought I was having a miscarriage, but part of me thought that if I did, all of my problems would be over. As for feelings about her while I was pregnant—I don't recall having any. I thought when she kicked, etc., that it was exciting, but I didn't have deep mother instincts. Basically my feelings were, "It's just you and me, kid." I considered us both to be victims. Kind of like the bond between hostages.

My feelings didn't change much during the pregnancy. As it

progressed, I continued to deny them. I just kept pretending we were a happy little family. The hardest thing I had to deal with were the times I would have to face the fact that this really wasn't Joe's baby. I suppose the best thing I felt was that I was doing everything that I thought I could for this baby.

After I had the baby, I wasn't aware that I had any negative feelings from the rape. Looking back, I see that I went into a state of depression. My interest in sex was gone. It repulsed me to have my husband touch me. When we did have sex, I quietly cried myself to sleep. I had tried to convince myself that the rape never happened. Then I would look at her and realize yes, it must have happened.

Joe's attitude changed. He constantly reminded me that she wasn't his baby. He began to doubt that I was raped. I began to have an eating disorder (binging & starving) that I still battle. Eventually, Joe and I divorced and I remarried a man named Michael.

For many years, I didn't think I had negative feelings related to the rape. But one day, after 15 years, my husband and I were at a gathering and I saw my rapist's brother. I couldn't say why, but I wanted to get out of there.

A few months later, Mike, the rapist, started attending our church. For two months I didn't recognize him. When I did, he was sitting in front of me. I wanted to cry. I wanted to beat him up side the head.

The feelings flooded in. My husband, Michael, listened to me talk, talk, talk, and cry, cry, cry, sometimes into the night. After a week of this I felt light and cleansed. I think that I had finally faced and dealt with my feelings and that God healed the wounds.

After that first week, I had no problems with him going to our church. He realized who I was, but seemed to have forgotten the rape. My husband, Michael, had a hard time dealing with everything. So our pastor went to Mike to suggest a couple of other churches that he should try. He wanted to know why. When the pastor told him that I had said that he had raped me, he went into a rage. He said I was a liar and that it was a mutual thing.

A couple of months later I talked to him. I retold him everything that happened that day when he raped me. He started to cry and he said, "I am a rapist!" I wonder how many men have raped women and later convinced themselves that they didn't. I feel, if possible, it would be good for a lot of rape victims if they could face their rapist.

I had told Beth the circumstances of her conception when she was almost 13. I don't think it's always best to tell them. In our case she knew that her father, Joe, didn't treat her very good and she couldn't stand him. She is also the kind of person that is strong and seems to be able to handle a lot, and I was afraid that she would hear it somewhere else. Probably if I had to do it a second time, I don't know if I would have told her Mike's name. Mike and Beth keep in contact on the phone. I'm not sure if that's the best, but they seem to really care for each other.

In some ways, I feel fortunate that I know Beth's biological father. I see very little negative characteristics that she shares with him. His negative characteristics are alcoholism, drug dependency, unreliability, and he's somewhat of a phony. Beth, on the other hand, is the opposite in these areas. What they do share is that they are both charming, outgoing, popular, and very ambitious.

My family didn't find out about the rape for nearly 14 years. I told my sister first. Surprisingly, I don't remember what she said, but she was very supportive. After a lot of encouragement from my sister and my husband, Michael, I finally told my mother. I was so scared, I was shaking all over.

Her first response was to chew me out for not telling her the truth in the beginning. After a few minutes she stopped and told me how sorry she was for the things she had said to me over the years. She said that she was proud of how well I had taken care of Beth, especially since I was so young and because of the things I had gone through. We talked and cried till two a.m.

When she told my dad, he didn't say much but she said he couldn't sleep all night. They don't say much about it now. It's probably pretty obvious that I don't want to talk about it with them. One time my mom called me, from work, to tell me that my dad had called her to tell me that there was a program on the 700 Club about rape victims. For some reason I felt annoyed. If anyone else had done that I would have been grateful.

I was relieved that everything was out in the open. But I was really relieved and surprised that they didn't blame me at all. Like I had already said, they wanted to help me, but I didn't want them to. The way they helped me the most was by showing me respect as a person.

Based on my experience, it is my belief that when women become pregnant after being raped they should be offered a loving and supportive environment. They need people to accept them and believe their story. They need to be counseled to recognize and deal with their feelings. I have had counseling with two psychologists and two pastors, none of whom knew how to deal with rape victims that conceived.

There is no doubt in my mind that abortion should be discouraged. Abortion is a terrible way of dealing with a pregnancy resulting from rape, although I suppose it is a way for people to ignore the victim and her needs. People seem to be afraid to think about rape. Rape is a big enough trauma to deal with. It's just that much more confusing when you throw more trauma like abortion into it.

I think that rape victims with pregnancies are discriminated against. People seem to think you're nuts to have a baby by a man who raped you. We are looked upon as being liars, or stupid.

I definitely think that adoption is usually the best answer. If I knew then what I know now, I would have given Beth up for adoption. She's had a crazy life. My first husband verbally abused her. I never have had, and still don't have, the maternal feelings for her that I have for my other kids. We're good friends and I so love her, but it's like we're sisters. I wish she could have had a more normal life.

If I had an opportunity to counsel a young girl or woman who became pregnant after a rape, I would try to let her see that she did nothing to deserve rape. I would tell her that the baby is no less a person just because of how it was conceived.

"When I defend the unborn I am defending my son's right to life."

—"Connie Sellers"

Twenty-eight years ago, "Connie" became pregnant as a result of rape. Although she chose to give birth to her child, she was in strong denial about his existence until she heard him cry. However, after she heard him cry, she realized how much she loved him. "Connie" placed her son for adoption. Today she has begun to search for him in the hope of being reunited with him.

Two weeks after my fifteenth birthday I was raped. Nine months later I bore a child.

I was a sophomore taking several difficult courses: Latin,

accelerated geometry, chemistry, etc. So I did not want to miss
school while my parents and sister went on a two-week vacation
in the middle of September. Anyway, in our church there was a
young newlywed couple living with the bride's family. They
agreed to stay with me during those two weeks so I wouldn't be
alone.

The Saturday before my family was to return, I was at home
alone cleaning and preparing the house for the much-awaited
return of my family when the husband returned alone. He
attacked me, tore my skirt at the waistband, and raped me. He
had no weapons—just his overpowering strength.

He could hold me down but he could not hold me still. I wig-
gled and scooted and at one point even got my legs crossed until
he rose in the air and kneed me in the groin. When he stopped,
I thought he had given up. I didn't realize he had finished. He
started crying and begging me to think of his wife.

Well, I didn't tell anyone, but it wasn't because I forgave him.
Nor was it because I was trying to spare his wife pain. I was simply too embarrassed. Besides, the only ones I could talk to had-
n't returned from vacation yet.

I didn't want anyone to know how I had been defiled. I hid
my torn skirt in the garage and cleaned up the blood. I felt dirty
and ashamed. I called my older married brother and asked if I
could spend the night with him. He knew I had been crying but
thought that I was just terribly homesick for my parents. By the
next day when my parents returned, I had decided it was just
better to never tell anyone and keep from having to talk about
something I didn't even want to remember.

A month of so later I started to wonder why I hadn't had a
period. I still didn't think I was pregnant. I thought the shock of
what had "almost" happened had thrown off my cycle.

Soon my belly began to develop a hard knot and I knew I was
pregnant, but I wanted to talk about what happened to me even
less now. I was still embarrassed but now I was also worried.
What would people think? Who would believe me?

I prayed for God to take it away. I would push on my belly
until it hurt to stop the growing bulge. I never considered it a
baby then. I started keeping my coat on indoors and finding a
pillow to hold when sitting. I was desperate and alone because
of my silence.

Finally, shortly after Christmas I told my mother that I had
been raped and thought I might be pregnant. I was almost four

months pregnant when I had my first gynecological exam. The doctor had to finish breaking the hymen in order to examine me. I had been able to avoid complete penetration.

The doctor told my brother that if we had come earlier he would have performed an abortion, but it was too dangerous this far into the pregnancy. The fact that abortion was then illegal didn't bother him, I guess.

My attacker at first denied ever touching me, then he said I had encouraged him. My family stood beside me, but everyone else seemed to doubt me. How could I have been raped if I was still alive? Why had I waited so long to say anything if I was so innocent? What about his wife? Didn't I think about the pain this caused her?

My parents went to an attorney who counseled my parents not to file charges and cause me further hurt. I went to a home for unwed mothers. The attacker agreed to pay for my stay, and I was put away in the home to hide.

They had a counselor in the home that saw the girls weekly, but she only saw me one time. She asked me to give her a blow-by-blow description of the rape and then she never talked to me again. With the other girls I imagined she discussed birth control, relationships with men, etc., but she didn't know what to say to me.

I was soon to be a mother but I had never had a date and had never had a grownup kiss. I needed counseling terribly. I needed someone to tell me sex wasn't always so painful, but could be beautiful in the union of a loving marriage, as God intended. I needed someone to tell me that all men were not to be feared. I needed to work through my feelings with a good Christian counselor, but neither my parents nor I thought to ask if any were available.

I seemed to be coping quite well. I knew God and did go to Him for help, but the denial was so strong that I asked to be blindfolded in the delivery room so I wouldn't have any visual memories of the birth. (Now any woman who has given birth knows that there must be pretty strong denial if you can go through labor and still deny there is a baby involved.)

I was able to deny my motherhood until I heard my baby's cry. Then I knew I was a mother. I kept on the blindfold but I wanted to know if he was healthy and what sex he was. I had a son.

I truly believe that God has given women hormones that

cause them to love their babies. Love them enough that they will
get up in the middle on the night and care for the baby's needs
at the expense of their own. By the next morning, I wanted to see
my baby, but I tried to resist. After two days I asked to see him,
feed him, hold him, and say goodbye.

They let us go into a room all to ourselves with a rocking
chair. I had never held such a small baby but it came naturally. I
fed him and held him for a very long time. I told him I loved him
but couldn't keep him. I told him that his birth was not his fault.
I told him to be a good little boy and make some family very
happy.

There is a scripture in Romans 8:28 about all things working
for the good of those who love God and are called according to
His purpose. Well, even after I went away from God because of
my lack of forgiveness, bitterness and rebellion, I never wished
that my son had never been born. He was the only good thing
about the rape. I loved that baby. I gave him away but I never
forgot him.

It gave me comfort to think of him making some other couple
happy. If I had taken his life there would have been no good.
Maybe God can use my testimony now for more good, to further
His kingdom and save the lives both of the unborn and the born.
I pray it is so.

Even if the rape victim was my own daughter, I would counsel her against abortion. Rape is hard enough to deal with, let
alone the guilt of murder.

Counseling for rape should include:

1. Learning to accept personal feelings of guilt. If there was
any encouragement—intentional or not, impure thoughts, etc.—
ask God's forgiveness, accept it, and forgive yourself.

2. Learning not to accept guilt from external sources; not to
take on guilt where there is innocence just because someone else
thinks you are guilty.

3. Learning to allow yourself to feel disgust and repulsion at
what has happened. Many years ago in secular counseling when
I allowed myself to feel that repulsion, I vomited until I thought
I would retch up my guts. Afterward I felt tremendous relief.

4. The BIG one: learning to forgive the attacker. This is not
mentioned in secular counseling and I think it's only possible
through God. This step is necessary for complete healing.

5. Belief that even though the attacker has taken something
(innocence, virginity) from you, God can restore and heal. God

is the answer!

I think that counselors need to hear and show rape victims that (1) I believe you (counselors should not play detective), (2) I love you (rejection and disgust hurt almost as much as the rape), and (3) God loves you. Secular counselors can only help bring health to a certain point. Through God we can come to forgiveness and wholeness—restored and new.

I don't know where my son is, but I recently sent out papers to begin a search for him. Wherever he is, I hope he knows God, and I hope he is involved in the pro-life movement.

"There have been many times when I have looked back grateful that no state legislature had provided an easy, instant answer of a free abortion for me."

—Lee Ezell

Lee is the mother of Julie Makimaa, whose story is found elsewhere in this book. The full account of Lee's story is found in her book, The Missing Piece. *The following is a letter she wrote to legislators opposed to allowing exceptions for abortion in the cases of rape and incest.*

An open letter to Representatives defending the unborn children conceived by sexual assault,

I would like to add my thanks to you for all your expressed compassion and concern for rape victims, much like myself. I was a virgin teenager, raped by a salesman passing through the place I worked. The experience of sexual assault was traumatizing enough, but to find myself pregnant was inconceivable. Born to alcoholic parents, I was told I was an "unwanted child." Now I was pregnant with an unwanted child. It wasn't fair.

I wound up going full-term with the pregnancy and gave birth to a baby girl in Los Angeles County Hospital. I never held her or saw her; she was adopted at birth. At that time, how could I have known she'd be the only child I would ever give birth to? How could I have known that one day we would be reunited, and that she and her family would bring such joy into our lives?

Never, in all the years after her birth, did I ever regret giving life to my daughter. However, there have been many times when I have looked back grateful that no state legislature had provided an easy, instant answer of a free abortion for me. I'm grateful because, at that time, I might have bought into the lie that an abortion would fix all my problems. But fortunately that temptation wasn't there.

Like any woman in a crisis pregnancy (whether married or unmarried, raped or not), a pregnant sexual assault victim might welcome an instant answer to her problem. But abortion is too permanent an answer to a temporary problem. The answer to problems resulting from rape is not abortion. Based on my years of experience, I don't believe abortion is an answer; it is an additional problem. Abortion may sound compassionate—even noble—but it isn't.

Providing an instant abortion for a woman in trauma may sound desirable to her at the time. But we all know that it is easy to make terrible decisions, especially when we are under emotional stress, such as recovering from a rape.

For a woman who is depressed, sniffing cocaine gives instant relief. For a woman overwhelmed by her problems, drinking may be instant relief. But these answers only lead to further problems, just as abortion also sets a woman up for future problems. Invariably, this "abortion answer" is offered without full disclosure of its potential impact.

I agree that in the case of rape, some drastic action should be taken. But I believe that punitive action should be taken against the rapist, not against another innocent victim of his violence: the child conceived. Why should the baby receive the death penalty for the violence of the father?

Since the release of my book about my own experience, *The Missing Piece* (Bantam Books, 1988), I have met probably a hundred other folks who, like my own beautiful daughter, announce themselves to be the result of either rape or incest. In every case, similar to my own Julie, I have found these people to be emotionally stable individuals who are so grateful they had the opportunity to live without an instant answer wiping out their lives. They all agree it does not matter how they began, but what they have become.

As you glance at the face of Julie, I hope you will think of her, and my experience, as you vote to refuse the easy instant answer of abortion for rape and incest victims.

Sincerely,
Lee Ezell

"Through our children we begin to see more clearly what love and sacrifice are all about. To give life is to receive life in all its fullness."

—Cindy Speltz

Having been raised in an abusive, chaotic household, Cindy was raped by a neighbor and became pregnant. Kicked out of the house by her alcoholic father, she was left jobless, penniless, homeless, uneducated and alone. Yet she managed to overcome these seemingly insurmountable odds in order to have and raise her daughter, Jenni. Today Cindy sees her daughter as a special gift from God to help her heal and truly experience the joy of a life released from shame and fear.

In late August of 1974, all the odds were against me, and then some. That night I became pregnant through an acquaintance rape. Not knowing at the time that is what I had experienced, I kept it to myself out of fear and shame.

Three months passed before I learned I was "with child." About that same time, I was kicked out onto the streets late one winter night by my extremely violent alcoholic father. I had not washed the dishes in the sink, so he went into a rage and started flinging his belt strap around at me once again. Then he told me to get out of his house. I began walking down a lonely, dark country road towards town with only a few clothes in a paper bag and a big secret—my pregnancy.

There I was, facing the world, forced into the dark of the night unprepared. All I could do at that moment was put one foot in front of the other and continue down the path of darkness. My journey into the night made me fully aware that I was homeless, jobless, motherless, penniless, uneducated, pregnant, and alone at the age of 18.

In the eyes of the world I was the perfect candidate for an abortion. Soon enough I would be devoured by advice from "well-meaning" people urging me to abort, pitting me against my unborn infant, giving me every indication that they disapproved of me carrying my child to term—using phrases like, "You can't be a mother," and "You know what you have to do." I even heard my own relatives prompting me to abort—including my father's mother.

One night I received a phone call at my girlfriend's apartment, where I was temporarily being allowed to sleep on her couch. It was him—the biological father of my unborn baby, the man who had raped me. He had heard through the grapevine that I was pregnant. He spoke sharply to me, treating me as if I were the offender, saying, "You'd better get an abortion! You'd better not tell anyone; leave me out of it! Get an abortion right now!"

I just said quietly and sadly, "You are denying this baby's life, and you are denying me." I hung up the phone feeling numb, experiencing the ultimate rejection on behalf of my defenseless and totally innocent baby. I knew first hand what it was like to be completely rejected by one's own parents.

You see, I was raised as a victim of violence. I was a slave to fear. I was the eldest child of a woman who had committed suicide by hanging herself when I was twelve years old. I had no focus in life except thinking about how to survive, how to stay alive from one day to the next, living under the fear and oppression of an alcoholic father who beat us daily without mercy. There was not one day in my life that I ever felt safe in my father's presence. I knew what abandonment, neglect, abuse, and exploitation was; I had lived it. The unbearable part was having to see my six younger siblings endure my father's violence every day we were under his influence. I saw everything through the eyes and heart of a lost child. I lived on the verge of despair.

I was now four and a half months along and I could feel my baby fluttering in my womb. I stayed awake past midnight on the couch, feeling quite restless. It was a freezing Minnesota winter night. As the reality of my situation began to set in after months of numbness, I had to face the fact that I had no plans for my future and no one to turn to. My mind turned to the night I had conceived this child.

It was very late and I had gone up to bed in my father's house. I remember throwing on my nightgown and falling into bed, feeling so exhausted that I immediately faded into a deep sleep. Then, in the dark of the night, I heard a squeak. I recognized it as the sound of my closet door being opened.

Although I could not see a thing, I just assumed it was my younger brother pulling a prank on me, trying to spook me. So I laid still and ignored the noise, not reacting. When a figure emerged from the closet and began to approach me, I became a bit more alert. As the person entered my bed I was very startled, recognizing him as a neighbor I knew from high school. As he began to "have his way with me," I froze up, paralyzed in fear. I do remember turning my head toward the door wanting to cry out, but there was no one to help me. Tears just started to stream down my face, dripping into my left ear. I was too afraid to speak beyond a whispered, "No."

I feared death. I feared my father's brutal beatings. I truly believed that I would be killed if anyone found out. I remembered seeing a butcher's knife in my father's hand, knowing he would be willing to use it. I saw death, so I did nothing. I just took it. Afterwards the neighbor just slipped away into the dark. To this day I have no idea how he got into the house. How long was he in my closet? Not even knowing that what he had done was against the law, I told no one what had happened to me.

Now this night, still feeling restless as I lay on the couch, I glanced up at the window where beautiful blue moonbeams were spilling in. I got up and walked into the veil of moonlight, gazing at the glorious full moon. Suddenly, I was filled with fear. I could hear a voice saying, "You might as well get rid of it. Just get rid of it!" I knew at once what it meant, and in anguish I placed my hands over my stomach, as if to protect my unborn baby. Then, at that very instant, I felt a peaceful presence that seemed to cut right through the shadows of the room, and a clear, gentle voice spoke to my heart: "This infant is sacred and of God. This child is destined for great good."

At the time, I did not understand what these words meant. But after going over my due date by three weeks and going through 29 hours of labor, I gave birth to a precious baby girl whom I named Jennifer. At seven pounds, four ounces, with blue eyes and dark hair, she was perfect in my eyes—so tiny, so vulnerable. As she was placed in my arms and I kissed her cheek, I knew in my heart of hearts that she belonged to God. I knew she was a sacred gift.

As my future and my daughter's future have unfolded, we have come to know more fully what that simple message of truth that I heard that winter night meant in our lives. My daughter's life is a testimony of great good. She has touched many lives in untold ways in her 24 years, and we are certain that God has a divine plan and purpose for every human being He creates. We are all sacred and of God, made in his image and likeness. Every single child ever conceived is destined for great good!

My daughter's identity is not to be found in the frail characteristics of her biological parents. Her identity is in being a child of God. Jennifer is the link that reconnected me to God. She was the gift that brought me out of fear and darkness into the Light of authentic Love. Children are the signature of life, written by the very hand of God.

During my pregnancy, I was completely stripped and void of every single resource. There was not one person to cling to or depend on. I was drowning in darkness, constantly aware of my helpless state. Yet I had one magnificent secret gift, a hidden treasure that only God knew. A gift of immense value that went beyond any measure or comprehension. That gift was the flourishing life of my unborn baby.

In accepting the wonderment of this little one, I was brought to the light of a hope that I never knew before her existence. In the anticipation of her birth, I received the grace, faith and trust I needed to strengthen my soul.

Through the eyes and hearts of our children we begin to see more clearly, with a deeper sense of the mystery of life and of God, what love and sacrifice are all about. To give life is to receive life in all its fullness.

Don't you see? God's heart loved me so much, He gave me the gift of Jennifer. And He loved her so much, that He gave her the title, Child of God!

CHAPTER SIX

TESTIMONIES OF CHILDREN CONCEIVED IN RAPE

"The circumstances of my conception are not talked about very much . . . It doesn't bother me to know or to talk about how I was conceived."

—"Beth Bailey"

Beth is the daughter of Sharon "Bailey," whose story was described earlier. She learned the circumstances of her conception when she was 13. She was 16 at the time this was written. In what is perhaps an unusual case, Beth knows her natural father and with her mother's consent, she is trying to establish a relationship with him.

My name is Beth and I am 16 years old. I am the daughter of a woman who was raped at the age of 16. My mother was invited by my father to his house to meet one of his friends. It was then that they went upstairs and my mother was assaulted. Later she found out she was pregnant.

My mother, feeling scared and alone, told her fiancé about the rape and her pregnancy, and they decided together that they would marry and tell people that I was their child. My mother and stepfather thought that we would all be a happy family, and that it was best to hide the truth about the assault.

As I grew up, my mother and father's love for each other began to fade. My father began to accuse her of lying about the rape. Like so many other assault victims, she was being punished by the distrust and lack of support from people who were closest to her.

The hardest thing for her and me was how my "dad" treated me. At first it wasn't a problem but as I grew older he would favor my brother, his natural son. He would insinuate that I was worthless and stupid. A few years later my mother and father divorced.

I first found out that I had been conceived in rape when I was 13. My mother sat down with me and told me the story of the events that led up to her pregnancy. When I was first told about

the assault, I was very confused. At 13, I didn't really understand what all this meant. I didn't know what to think.

But I did have a desire to meet my natural father. All I could
think about was meeting him. A few years later I did!

The circumstances of my conception are not talked about very
much. Some people think that it is a big secret and they don't
want to hurt me. I wish that they would talk about it more. It
doesn't bother me to know or to talk about how I was conceived.

I feel that if a woman becomes pregnant by rape or incest she
should have the baby, and if it is necessary, release the child for
adoption so that the baby will have both a mother and a father
to raise him or her. I would very strongly discourage abortion.
It is the taking of a baby's life. The child should not be the one
to be punished. I also don't feel that abortion is a helpful way
out.

I have had the chance of meeting my natural father and have
gotten to know him a little. We have tried to have a relationship,
but he has a lot of problems in his life, including alcoholism, that
he is trying to deal with. We talk on the phone quite a bit. He
thinks I'm wonderful, and vice versa. But I never know what to
expect from him. He is very irresponsible, and obviously isn't
right in the head. Still, I am thankful that I had the chance to
meet my natural father and to know that he is sorry for the pain
that he caused my mother.

Finding out that I was conceived in rape has not influenced
my life much. I feel that children like me have a right to live, and
to know the circumstances of our conceptions. I feel that being
a child who resulted from rape or incest is nothing to be
ashamed of.

I hope that my story will be an example to show that abortion
is not a helpful way for a woman to deal with a pregnancy that
results from rape or incest.

**"I like the passage in Psalm 13, verse 6, that says: '. . . I will
sing to the Lord for He has been good to me.' Truer words cannot be found for my life."**

—**Rob "Smith"**

*Rob's birth mother was raped in 1957 and kept the circumstances of
her son's conception a secret for more than 30 years. It wasn't until*

*Rob began a search for her and located her that his mother told the
story of how she had become pregnant. Even though he still has not
been able to meet his mother in person, he is thankful that she chose to
give him life and place him in a loving home.*

My birth mother was 19 years old and a nursing student in
1957. She was an only child and lived with her parents; her
father was an Irish immigrant. I have no information in regard
to whether or not she told anyone about being sexually assaulted at the time of this incident, or how in fact she discovered she
was pregnant. The information regarding my adoption stated
that she did not believe she was pregnant until she went into
labor, but knowing that she was a nursing student somehow
casts a bit of doubt on that statement. It was noted however, that
she did not develop a "forward show" like many other women
and that this, they felt, may have been a contributing factor to
her denial.

Her own mother transported her to the hospital when she
went into labor and, once again relying on statements in the
adoption information, displayed what we would call today a
"real attitude!" The social worker assigned to the case noted that
the mother and daughter did not share a good relationship with
each other and that the mother was very concerned about protecting the family reputation. It would seem also that neither my
birth mom or her mother informed her father of the true nature
of her hospitalization and that funds were manipulated to pay
the hospital bill without arousing his curiosity. There was also
an obvious urgency on their part to have the adoption handled
in as rapid a manner as the legal system would permit, and no
one felt it in anyway prudent to inform my birth father of the situation.

I consider myself fortunate that I have known from an early
age that I was adopted. Indeed, even in childhood there arose
several situations in which it was disclosed to me by other than
family members. As a child I was diagnosed with learning dis-
abilities and was sent for various tests and evaluations with a
series of doctors, therapists, social workers and other professionals. It was during one such evaluation and exam that the
doctor began to recite his notes into the dictaphone and made
mention of "the patient's mother water skiing two weeks before
the birth which may have produced a pre-birth injury." I knew
that my adoptive mother did not participate in that sport so I

asked the doctor, "Hey, is that about me?" He was shocked that I was still in the room and immediately shut off the machine. But from that moment on I knew that sometime in my life I would want to meet that water-skiing lady.

I made two half-hearted attempts to search for my birth mother when I was between the ages of 18 and 25, but did not pursue a search fully until the fall of 1991. My search lasted a year but I was able to make the first contact four months after affiliating with a local adoptee search-support group. The phone call was made by my search assistant and while my birth mom acknowledged much of the information we had found out about her, she denied any knowledge of me or my birth.

Mind you, at this point we did not know the facts about the assault. We surmised at this point that maybe she felt my search assistant was me and did not know how to handle that. So I asked the president of our group if she would mind making a contact. She is a birth mother herself and we felt she would be an excellent peer for my birth mom. Once again my birth mom denied any knowledge of my birth or birth relatives. This really perplexed me because I've always felt that it must be impossible to deny the reality of having given birth.

I discovered in my search that I had three half-siblings, so I began to accumulate data on where they were so that contact could be maintained with at least one of them. As I was planning my strategy at work one evening a coworker inquired what I would say to them once I found them. I have to admit that threw me for a loop because I had not yet thought that part out. I realized that it would be traumatic for them to hear about me and that it would put me up for questions that I couldn't answer.

So I decided instead that my birth mom needed to hear from me directly. She had the right to know that the two previous contacts had been made because I requested that they be made. She had the right to know that the phone calls were not someone's idea of a cruel joke. She had the right to know that I was alive and in need of medical and other personal information. And she had the right to phone, correspond, or in some other way keep in contact with me if it was her desire to do so.

So I wrote my birth mom a letter providing her with my current address and phone number. I explained as best I could why I had searched for her and that I would appreciate any medical-genetic information that she could provide. I also provided her with the names and phone numbers of the two people who had contacted her in the event that she felt as though she could not speak or write to me directly. As it turned out, this was the option she chose to use.

She contacted the president of the search-support group shortly after receiving the letter. In an emotional conversation she disclosed that the contacts had been upsetting to her because she was finding she needed to cover them up to her family. She said that apart from her own mother no one else in the family was aware of the events of 1957. And then came the big bomb. She admitted to another person for the first time in her life that she had conceived me during a sexual assault—what we refer to today as a date rape. She had kept this secret for more than 30 years!

As you can imagine, this kind of blew me out of the water. I had no idea that this was even a possibility. But it did help me to see my birth mom as a victim and not the "bad girl" or "tramp" image that is sometimes associated with unwed mothers. Also I'm glad that this secret is now in the open because of the large numbers of services that are now available to victims of sexual assault. From what I understand they do not care if the assault happened 30 seconds or 30 years ago.

This revelation has made me even more aware of the mystery of God's grace. You see, not only did my birth mom admit to the rape, but she also stated that I should consider myself lucky in that, had the laws of the 50s been as they are today, she would have aborted! So I praise God because "I am fearfully and wonderfully made, and indeed all my days were planned before one of them came to be."

As far as my birth mom is concerned I feel much sympathy for her and the lack of support that was available when she needed it. I admire her ability to finish her nurses' training and stay in that field her entire life. Even with all the information I have I would still like to see her someday. Why? Because she's my mom and without her (and God) I wouldn't be here today.

As far as my biological father is concerned my opinion of him is that he is a criminal. Yet I want to reserve judgment on him because I have not heard his side of the story. Most likely he is in dire need of education on the issue of rape. I feel as though perhaps he may have felt that his action was a normal part of a dating relationship. That's not to say I excuse his action. Before there can be repentance there has to be an acknowledgment that a transgression has taken place . . . Of course this is all conjecture on my part. At this time, however, I have no immediate plans to search for him. If a relationship is going to develop with either of my birth parents I would prefer it to be with my birth mom who brought me into the world.

Because I have only very recently come by this knowledge (that I was conceived in a rape) I have not experienced any ramifications socially or in my family. At this time the word has not yet gotten out on the family grapevine.

Knowing myself, however, I feel that I have not inherited one iota of negative or evil traits because of my biological father's actions. In fact, just the opposite is true. I have loved the Lord since childhood and have taken great joy in serving in His house. I have remained faithful to my wife during our 13 years of married life and was a virgin up to our wedding night. So anyone looking for deviant tendencies will have to look somewhere else.

When a woman or girl finds herself pregnant due to sexual assault the first matter must be to contact the law enforcement authorities. Rape is a crime and I feel that much of the coping process for the victim must begin with the legal enforcement of justice. Secondly, she should be put in contact with a strong support group. Because the legal process may not relieve her anxiety, she must have a support system for her emotional well-being.

Under no circumstances should the victim consider an abortion! I feel that would only focus the anger of the crime against another innocent victim. Because I was adopted I feel that adoption is a very loving thing for a victim to do for her child, yet it may not be what every victim desires.

I remember several a years ago a tract was being circulated by a pro-life group that had the reader assume the role of a social worker faced with job of authorizing or denying funds for abortions. Several "hard cases" where presented and the reader was told to select which of the cases would be granted the funds for an abortion. The catch was that in each case if the abortion was approved, you wound up aborting a person who achieved high acclaim in his or her life.

Drawing from my personal experience I have to say that I am offended by that tract now. For while I have not achieved any real local or national fame, I have none the less been an important person in the lives of many people. Let's not worry about what Einstein or Beethoven we are killing but what biology teacher, police officer, emergency medical technician, Sunday school teacher, or pastor is being killed. It is the worst human tragedy in the history of the earth that we have killed and are killing countless "common" people with common aims and desires.

I am 35 years old, married 13 years, and the father of three children. I am a high school graduate who has pursed a career as an emergency medical technician. I have been active in the Lord's house since my youth. I have been a youth group officer, sung and still sing in the choir, been a soloist, and recently completed lector training. The realization of how I entered this world has increased my desire to serve the Lord as fully as I am able. I like the passage in Psalm 13, verse 6, that says: ". . . I will sing to the Lord for He has been good to me." Truer words cannot be found for my life.

"After all, it does not matter how we began in life. What matters is what we will do with our lives."

—Julie Makimaa

Julie was placed for adoption in a Christian home. As a young married woman, Julie searched for her birth parents, at least in part to witness to them about her faith in Christ. After a long search she found her mother, Lee Ezell, who herself was involved in a Christian ministry. But she also learned that she had been conceived during rape. Learning this truth has motivated Julie to take up the cause of "the least of God's children," those conceived by sexual assault and considered expendable by society. She founded Fortress International to represent the concerns and needs of pregnant sexual assault victims and their children.

I was adopted as a child by a family with two sons who wanted a daughter. When I was five, my parents started attending an Assembly of God church. There as a young girl I learned the stories of the Bible. We attended almost every service and if the doors were open you could find us there.

One Sunday night during a worship service I went forward to ask Jesus to come into my heart and to forgive me of my sins. Salvation through Jesus was a normal thing to me. Everyone at church was saved and I knew it was the right thing to do.

I was just a little girl but I knew that I had made a very important decision. Just to make sure I did it correctly, I raised my hand on a couple of other occasions at church when there was a call to accept Christ.

When I was seven, I was told by a girlfriend that I was adopted. I did not know exactly what that meant but knew that it was different from my other friends. I never thought that my parents loved me any less than my older brothers, but I knew that I was unique. I never really thought about my natural parents too much, but I sometimes wondered if I had ever unknowingly seen them or passed them on the street.

As I grew older, I began to see the importance of God in my family's life. I had grown up attending church and always felt that I would some day become a missionary, or travel and tell people about God. I remember one day while I was sitting in church an older lady sitting beside me bent down and told me that God was going to use my life in a very special way. I didn't know what to think, but I have never forgotten the words she spoke to me.

In 1980 I met a very special man who was a Christian, and we felt that the Lord had brought us together. The following year we married and moved to a small town in northern Michigan. I think that this was the time when I started to put into practice all of the things that I had learned as a child. I could no longer rely on my parents to show me the correct way, but I had to take the responsibility myself for my relationship with Christ. During the next three years I began to see how the Lord was working in my life.

After our marriage, I received my adoption papers from my parents. I felt a desire to begin searching for my birth parents. I wanted the opportunity to share with them my faith in Christ and salvation, so that no matter what they faced, they would find comfort in the fact that God does not forget us, but that all things work together for good to them that love God.

I am thankful that my adoptive parents gave me their support as I began my search for my birth mother. Their support meant a lot to me, and I was relieved that they did not feel threatened by my search. I felt that my adoptive parents were my "real" parents, and that would never change no matter what, and that there could never be anyone that could take their place.

My husband and I began to grow in our relationship with God. We felt that He had guided us to become involved in three specific areas: abortion, politics, and especially prayer for our country. As we began to participate in these areas, we could have never imagined what the Lord was preparing us for.

During this time some verses became very special and personal to us, such as Proverbs 24:11-12: "Rescue those who are unjustly sentenced to death; don't stand back and let them die. Don't try to disclaim responsibility by saying you didn't know about it. For God, who knows all hearts, knows yours, and he knows you knew! And he will reward everyone according to his deeds."

After three-and-a-half years of searching I found a couple that my natural mother had stayed with when I was born. After receiving my letter they called my mother and informed her of my search.

The next morning I received a call from my natural mother, Lee Ezell. It was numbing to speak with her, my mother whom I never met, for the first time. As we cautiously talked, I could not stop myself from pondering all the questions that I wanted to ask. I did not know if I would ever speak with her again, and I knew that I wanted to tell her about my belief and relationship with God.

I told her about myself and some of my interests. She had to be aware by now that most of my conversation was fixated on my involvement with church. I thought this was a good time to find out if she had ever heard about Jesus. I was shocked as she began to tell me about her relationship with God, her women's speaking ministry, radio program, and writing her first Christian book. Lee had already been a follower of the Savior!

I had always thought that God needed to use me to save my natural parents. I never considered that they may already know Jesus. It's strange how sometimes we think we need to help God out, like He can't do things without us.

Lee and I excitedly made plans to meet only eight weeks from our first phone call. It was bizarre to think that I was really going to meet her. Would she be like I had imagined? What would she think of me? I hoped that she would like me.

After searching for nearly four years, I was enthusiastic about our reunion. I was going to see her face to face! It took a while to get used to the idea; it was almost unbelievable. And she was a Christian. Things had worked out so much better than I could ever have imagined. God gives us such good gifts.

One afternoon as my husband Bob and I sat at home, we received a call from Lee's husband Hal. When I answered the phone and he asked to speak with Bob, I knew something was wrong.

I immediately thought that Lee had changed her mind about the reunion. As I listened to Bob, I was having difficulty piecing together the conversation, but I could tell that it wasn't good. They wanted to tell him first so that he could decide whether or not to tell me. The circumstances of my conception were not unblemished, and if it were to take place today, my father probably would be put in jail.

At that time Bob and I did not know if Lee had become pregnant as a result of rape or incest, but I knew either situation would have been very devastating for Lee. I was sure that our reunion was off.

This was a time when I had to decide whether or not I really believed the things I had been taught as a little girl. I had to believe that God was in control of the situation. I could not figure out why He allowed me to find her under these conditions. I knew that God made the decisions about life, but I had to go back and remind myself that it didn't matter about my conception. God had a plan, and He was my real Father, and I was born because of His love, not by accident.

I wondered if Lee and I were really meant to get together. I felt that because of the circumstances Lee could not bear the emotional stress of seeing me. I was afraid that my finding her would bring back difficult memories of what happened, and I had never wanted to cause problems for her.

I was overwhelmed to get a call from Lee asking if everything was still on for our reunion. She told me that the assault was in her past and that she had been healed from that experience. She still wanted to meet me. God was still in the driver's seat!

As we met for the first time in a Washington, D.C. hotel, I was numb. There were so many emotions of excitement, fear, and happiness!

As we got over the first few minutes of excited tension, my husband Bob said the words that expressed how truly important our reunion was. Bob told Lee how grateful he was that she did not have an abortion, but that she gave of herself for a few months, allowing me to share a lifetime with him. It was a very special moment.

It was amazing to think that we were together after twenty-one years. Later that night Lee and Hal told us how she had been raped and became pregnant with me. As we talked about my feelings about knowing the circumstances of my conception, and Lee's feelings about our reunion, we knew that God had brought us together and had a special plan for all of us. Bob encouraged Lee to write a book about her experiences and our reunion, and for it to be an example about how God works in our lives. Not long afterwards, she did. It's entitled *The Missing Piece*. That means me!

It was time to leave Washington and go back home, but I never could have imagined how much my life was going to change. In the car on the long drive back to northern Michigan, Bob and I felt that the Lord had been preparing us for something, and that His plans would take us away from our home.

Our involvement in pro-life activities increased. In the past we had never made a decision about pregnancies that resulted from rape or incest. But now we knew what Christ would teach in these cases. He loves all of His children, even those conceived in the worst of circumstances; and He will take care of His children if only we trust in His care. After all, it does not matter how we began in life. What matters is what we will do with our lives.

How could we tolerate abortion in these "hard cases," especially after knowing that I was the result of such a pregnancy? I knew that if God was in control of my life and that if He was still working things out for our good, then I had to believe that He could do it for others like Lee and I. So, I began to speak out on these issues . . . that every preborn child deserves the right to live and that abortion is wrong. "Before I formed you in the womb I knew and approved of you [as My chosen instrument], and before you were born I separated and set you apart, consecrated you, and I appointed you a prophet to the nations." (Jeremiah 1:5)

When this verse in Jeremiah speaks to me, I know that God has a special plan and job for my life. It's something only I can do; some person only I can touch.

No, I am not going to be a prophet like Jeremiah. But I can speak out for the unborn children like myself who were conceived by sexual assault.

Many times I felt like Moses, knowing that I am not a good speaker and that there were so many other people that could do a much better job. But I realized that if I believed, God would give me the words to say when I needed His help.

Through my life I have seen over and over the faithfulness of God to do what He said He would do. Now I feel that the Lord has led me to work specifically to help women who have become pregnant as a result of sexual assault, and to work with children who have been conceived in rape or incest.

Women who become pregnant through assault need to know that it was not their fault, and that they are not dirty because of it. They are innocent, just like their children who are conceived in rape. Many women who carry these children to term fall in love with them. There is also adoption for women who feel that they are not prepared to raise a child.

Knowing God and wanting to do the things that He has planned for me has affected every area of my life. How I dealt with my adoption, who I married, my reaction to learning I was conceived in rape, and now my work with women and children. I believe that if I had not been raised in a Christian home, my life today would be much different. It is never too late for someone to ask Jesus into their life, and to begin to accomplish the special things that God has planned for their lives.

There have been so many times when I have failed to do the things I know I should have done, and many times I have let the Lord down, but it is great to know that no matter how many times I mess up, He is there ready to forgive me when I ask.

I was given the greatest gift by my parents that any parent can give to a child. It was not having all the toys I wanted, it was being raised attending church and learning the truth about God's love and salvation through his son Jesus Christ. The greatest gift a parent can give is the gift of passing on the knowledge of a true relationship with God. I believe that this gift, above all others, has affected every area of my life, and will continue to for the rest of my existence.

Thank you, Mom and Dad, for raising me in a home where I could develop a relationship with God. I am not only grateful for myself, but also for my children who are being raised the same way. It is exciting to see them learn the stories of the Bible as I did, and I look forward to seeing them follow the wonderful, secret plan that God has for their lives.

Thank you, Lee, for giving me life and the chance to know God, and for praying that I would go to a Christian home. I am grateful for my life. Thank you for the gift of life which I can share with my children and grandchildren, and maybe even my great-grandchildren. In protecting my life, despite the hardships it caused you, you saved not just me, but countless generations to come.

Thank you, my Father in Heaven. Your ways are mysterious,

and sometimes hard to endure, but they are always fruitful. Help us all to trust in and cherish Your gift of life.

SECTION III

INCEST AND ABORTION

CHAPTER SEVEN

THE DESTRUCTION OF INNOCENCE

David C. Reardon, Ph.D.

"Rape and incest . . ." Hand in hand, these two words were the Trojan horse of the abortion rights movement. But as with rape, abortion proponents have appealed to the public's aversion to incest to gain support for their cause while ignoring the real needs of the victims. Abortion was simply *presumed* to be the best solution for pregnant incest victims.

Pro-abortionists suggest that through abortion we can "help" these embarrassing victims of our sick society. We can destroy the "unclean" offspring of sexual perversions. But like rape, there is no psychiatric evidence, or even any theory, to support the idea that abortion will help a pregnant incest victim. Abortion is simply convenient for everyone else, especially the perpetrator.

Setting aside these paternalistic attitudes, we must ask what pregnant incest victims themselves want. Studies show that they almost always desire to keep their babies. Those who do abort generally do so unwillingly, usually under pressure from the impregnating relative who is seeking to cover up his crime.[1]

The reasons why incest victims want to keep their children are as complex as the issue of incest itself. Some see the pregnancy as an opportunity to expose and escape the incestuous relationship. For others, the unborn child represents a chance to establish a truly loving relationship, as opposed to the exploitive one in which they are entangled. Still others see giving birth as a chance to show their maturity and "win" their parents' respect.

INCEST AS A FAMILY PATHOLOGY

Incest can only be understood as a family pathology. The relationships between the husband, wife, and children are often strange and twisted. One researcher put it well when she said: "Reading the literature on incest is like trudging through a sewer."[2] Every member of a family touched by incest is embroiled in psychological turmoil, though the young victim is undoubtedly the most vulnerable and confused.

Incest can take many forms, so making generalizations about incest is a poor substitute for studying it closely. Due to space limitations, however, we can only offer a brief overview of "typical" incest patterns that illustrate some of the underlying problems involved in an incest pregnancy.

Most cases of incest involve the male guardian and a teenage or even a pre-teenage girl. Though the perpetrator is frequently the girl's natural father, incestuous relationships with stepfathers or the mothers' common law husbands are much more common. Incest with other men, such as uncles, brothers, or cousins, appear to represent only a minority of cases.[3]

Frequently the incestuous adult will begin to sexually "train" the girl for use at a very young age, sometimes as early as seven or eight. He will continue the relationship until she runs away or marries, or until the incest is exposed to outside authorities and intervention takes place.

Offenders have various motives for engaging in incest. Some involve sexual perversions. Other perpetrators are drawn more by the inadequacies of their marital relationships or by their own sense of low self-esteem. Because the victim is ignorant and naive, the perpetrator sees in her an opportunity to obtain a sexual "conquest" in which he hopes to restore his sense of masculinity or exert a sense of authority, control, or dominance over women.

Power and control are key elements of incestuous relationships. For some perpetrators, sexual excursions with their daughter or step-daughter are an easy escape from marital problems. Because of her youth and dependency, it is easier to dominate and control his incestuously-trained daughter than to overcome conflicts with his wife.

In other cases, the incestuous act lacks any elements of manipulation and seduction and is indistinguishable from an act of violent rape. Such cases will almost always include intimidating threats if the "secret" is revealed.

In at least a few cases, the family pathology is so deeply entrenched, perhaps spanning several generations, that the young girl is seen as a sexual plaything by all the males in the family. She may be abused by her father, brothers, and cousins as well. In such cases, the girl may suffer in passive silence, accepting her abuse as "normal" because it is all she has ever known.

Obviously, the incest victim is manipulated by many psychological games of deceit and intimidation. Although she may never consent to the incest, she is made to feel obligated to submit to it. She is likely to feel guilty (often without understanding exactly why), isolated, afraid, and uncertain about how to change her circumstances. Though she may recoil from her father's advances and dread future repetitions of their sexual contact, it is also likely that she has a sincere love for her father and a strong need to be loved by him. Though she may find their sexual relationship confusing or even repulsive, at least she finds in it some sense of the attention and love she so desperately needs. Though she would much rather be a daughter than a sex-object, the latter form of attention is sometimes accepted as a meager substitute.

Daughters victimized by incest frequently feel that their mothers are bad mothers, and they may fear that they, too, will be bad mothers. They may feel estranged from their mothers and expect little support from the mother in escaping the incestuous relationship. Indeed, often the mother may actually be aware of the incest but will refuse to believe it or will fail to act. The daughter's attempts to hint at what is happening and to seek help are often rebuffed and ignored by her mother, who simply does not want to believe it.

Sometimes, such denial can be taken to extremes. In one case, the mother had repeatedly seen her nude husband in bed with her daughter during a two-and-a-half year period but ignored her "suspicions" until pregnancy occurred. In yet another case, where an incestuous pregnancy was ultimately reported by an outside party, the mother had simply "reassured her four daughters that father was merely trying to show affection by manipulating their breasts and vaginas."[4]

ABORTION AND THE CONSPIRACY OF SILENCE

Because it incorporates so many strained relationships, incest is usually shrouded in a "conspiracy of silence." The daughter is too ashamed to discuss it and doubts that there is any aid to be found; the mother denies what she doesn't want to believe; and, of course, the father seeks desperately to conceal it. All of them may know what is happening, but they will not even

admit it to each other, much less to the outside world. Until this
denial is overcome, breaking the incestuous pattern is impossible. Until the incest is exposed, it is unlikely that the family will
seek treatment.

The person who most wants out of the incestuous situation is
the victim, the daughter. Through friends, teachers, doctors or
relatives, she may eventually drop enough hints to arouse suspicion and action. Failing that, she may simply "wait it out"
until she is old enough to move away, or she may seek other
more immediate avenues of escape: running away, early marriage, or pregnancy.

Though the daughter wants out, it should be remembered
that she would prefer to break the incest pattern in a way which
would allow her to maintain or regain the love of her parents.
Pregnancy is an avenue which offers to fulfill both requirements.[5]

Abortion of an incestuous pregnancy not only adds to the
girl's guilt and trauma, but also frustrates her plans for escape
and attention. Abortion perpetuates the "conspiracy of silence"
by covering up the incest, or at least its results, and continues
the family pattern of denying reality. Indeed, in some cases
where the daughter maintains a positive attitude toward her
father, her feelings turn negative only when he insists upon an
abortion or denies his paternity, thus frustrating her attempts at
acceptance and escape. Although nearly half of all incestuous
fathers press for abortion if a pregnancy occurs, most daughters
are strongly opposed to it. Only a quarter of incest cases result
in the daughter submitting to abortion.[6]

Ready access to abortion increases the likelihood that incest
victims will continue to be abused by contributing to the conspiracy of silence. What else can we expect when minors are
offered abortions without any attempt to identify and prosecute
those who are guilty of incest or statutory rape?

Writing under the pseudonym "Mary Jean Doe," one feminist
writer who was sexually abused by her older brother and one of
his friends describes how "the system" ignores signs of abuse:

> About three or four months after the abuse began, I was late for a
> period . . . I turned to my Sunday School teacher for help. When I
> told her I thought I might be pregnant (at 12 years old), she did-
> n't even blink. She gave me a hug and said I should go to
> Planned Parenthood for a "rabbit test," that I should get one of
> my older brothers to take me and not tell my parents. She never

asked who the male partner was or why I was sexually active at that age.

So my older brother took me to Planned Parenthood . . . The whole visit was terrifying . . . No one expressed any dismay, concern, or even interest that a 12-year-old girl needed a pregnancy test. I heard a lot about 'being responsible' and 'taking control of my body.' Someone gave me a handful of condoms on the way out and made a joke about it being an assortment—red, blue, and yellow . . .

My older brother maintained a strong silence throughout the entire visit—no one asked him a single question.

Two days later I received a phone call telling me the test was positive and to come in the following Saturday with a sanitary napkin and a friend who could drive. The caller never used the word 'pregnant' or 'abortion.' I did not keep the appointment; my period started that evening . . .

It was not until three years later that I discovered, in a high school biology class . . . what intercourse was . . . I remember the feeling of horror that came over me as I realized I had been scheduled for an abortion . . .

The sexual attitude often championed by Planned Parenthood is a serious factor in preventing the discovery of sexual abuse of young people. Everyone around me seemed to accept as normal that a 12-year-old girl could and should be sexually active (so long as she is 'responsible'—remember to use a rubber!) And remember, too, who took me to Planned Parenthood—an older brother with an urgent interest in my having an abortion!

Abortion on demand, no questions asked, makes it easier for incest and child abuse to continue. Abortion for incest victims sounds compassionate, but in practice it is simply another violent and deceptive tool in the hand of the abuser.[7]

ABORTION'S IMPACT ON INCEST VICTIMS

Leaving aside the issue of the unborn child's right to live (valid though it is), abortion of an incestuous pregnancy is simply bad medicine. It carries psychological and physical risks which are especially high for adolescents, and even higher risks for adolescents who are forced into an abortion unwillingly. In addition, because the victim desires the pregnancy as a means to expose her circumstances, it is frequently not discovered or revealed until the second or even third trimester. In such cases, the health risks associated with an abortion are several times greater than those associated with most teenage abortions.[8]

Clearly, for the incest victim her primary emotional need is to have the incest stopped and to have access to family counseling. Rarely, if ever, does the pregnant incest victim desire an abortion. She simply does not see her baby as the problem; rather, it is the *incest* that is the problem. To her, the chief difficulties associated with her pregnancy are the negative reactions and rejection of those around her: her parents, family, friends, physician, and counselors.

Unlike pregnancies resulting from rape, most incest pregnancies are actually desired, at least at a subconscious level, in order to expose the incest. A study of girls with incestuous pregnancies showed that "problems in accepting the pregnancy and birth of the child seemed related more to the negative reaction of friends and other relatives and to tensions which developed between the parents or between mother and daughter as a result of the pregnancy."[9]

As Dr. Fred Mecklenburg notes, abortion in cases of incest is counterproductive: "Furthermore, the incestuous relationship requires psychiatric care. With proper management, the outcome of incest may not always be as traumatic as was previously believed . . . Incest is basically a family pathology. Treating it as such, there is evidence that there may be gain for all concerned when the family cooperates in treatment. Aborting an innocent unborn child will neither correct the pathology nor mend the hurts. The problem exists with or without pregnancy, with or without abortion."[10]

Dr. George Maloof goes further, insisting that abortion is counterproductive for incest victims because it represents a "further assault upon their sexual integrity." Childbirth allows incest victims to "take a step toward accepting responsibility for their sexual acts and thereby toward freedom from the self-destructive effects of both incest and abortion." He believes adoption should be strongly recommended in incest cases, so as to facilitate repair of what is already a severely torn family structure: "Only after having the child adopted can there be some assurance that this new life will not simply become part of the incestuous family affair. The family can be consoled by the knowledge that they have broken their incestuous pattern . . ."[11]

In conclusion, Dr. Maloof writes:

> If the only way we can help the [incest victims] is to kill their babies and take away their fathers, are we not taking away the people for whom she cares the most? If her mother rallies to her side only to get rid of her father and child, isn't the pattern of avoiding problems being perpetuated? . . . Are we reenacting the maternal rejection felt by the daughter which predisposed the incest situation, so that the daughter is dramatically demonstrating what she feels the mother has done to her? Are we indirectly killing the daughter who feels her child is an extension of herself?
>
> Whatever else we may be doing by an abortion of an incestuous pregnancy, we are promoting mental illness . . . Accepting the pregnancy can be the first step to accepting the incest and making the changes to alter the family pattern so that it can be more productive rather than withholding and destructive.[12]

Whenever a young adolescent in impregnated through incest, statutory rape, or juvenile sexual experimentation, it is likely that she will be strongly attached to the idea of having her child. It is true that a 12-year-old girl is unlikely to have a realistic expectation of the responsibilities of parenthood. It is also true that her love for the child may be shaped by an unrealistic fantasy about having a real-life "doll" to play with. But the fact that a young girl does not fully appreciate a child's impact on her life is no reason to ignore her feelings. It is certainly no excuse for forcing her into an unwanted abortion "for her own good."

It is precisely the young girl's attachment to her baby, whether realistic or unrealistic, which insures with 100 percent reliability that she will be traumatized by an abortion. To the young girl, the abortion is not an act of free will by which she is regaining her future. It is the destruction of her baby, her "baby doll" even. It is the destruction of her dream, the ripping away of her innocence.

Everyone can agree, in principle, that 12-year-old girls should not have babies. But once the 12-year-old is pregnant, the choice is not simply between having a baby or not having a baby. The choice is between having a baby and having an abortion. The choice is between having a baby or having a traumatic experience. Which would the young girl rather have? A baby or a traumatic surgery wherein she is forced to participate in the murder of her baby?

Abortion does not simply make the girl "unpregnant." It does not turn back the clock. It is a violent and intrusive procedure which inflicts physical and psychological trauma on women of all ages, especially on adolescents whose self-images are still developing. For the 12-year-old incest victim, abortion is another shattering blow to her view of herself as a person, a woman, and a mother. She will be bruised by this experience for the rest of her life.

Edith Young, a 12-year-old incest victim impregnated by her stepfather, writes 25 years after her child was aborted:

> Throughout the years I have been depressed, suicidal, furious, outraged, lonely, and have felt a sense of loss. I have felt, and at times still feel, that my mother and stepfather owe me something. What? I don't know. Maybe a sincere, 'I'm sorry.' Even if my daughter had been put up for adoption, instead of killed, some of the pain would not be present.

> Often I cry. Cry because I could not stop the attacks. Cry because my daughter is dead. And I cry because it still hurts. They say time heals all wounds. This is true. But it doesn't heal the memories, at least not for me.

> I've suffered many physical problems and continue to do so. Ever since the abortion, I've suffered chronic infections of my tubes, ovaries and bladder. The pains from my menstrual periods were nightmarish and continued from the time of my abortion until my partial hysterectomy in November 1982. In April of this year, I again had surgery. There was a growing, bleeding cyst on my left ovary. On my right side, there were a massive amount of adhesions and the ovary could not be found. Twenty-five years have gone by but the consequences of the abortion are still going on.

> As you can see, the abortion which was to 'be in my best interest' just has not been. As far as I can tell, it only 'saved their reputations,' 'solved their problems,' and allowed their lives to go merrily on.

> My daughter, how I miss her so. I miss her regardless of the reason for her conception. You see, she was a part of me, an innocent human being, sentenced to death because of the selfish sexual gratification of another and the need to 'save reputations.' She was a unique individual whose life was exterminated . . . How I miss her so.[13]

Portions of this article were previously published in Aborted Women, Silent No More *by David C. Reardon, Loyola University Press., 1987..*

NOTES

1. Dr. George Maloof, "The Consequences of Incest: Giving and Taking Life," *The Psychological Aspects of Abortion*, David Mall and Walter Watts, eds (Washington D.C.: University Publications of America, 1979) 73-110. Dr. Maloof's article is the primary source for all information used in this section on incest.

2. Meehan, "Facing the Hard Cases," *The Human Life Review*, Summer 1983, 25.

3. Ibid.

4. Maloof, "The Consequences of Incest," 76.

5. Ibid., 73-83. Also, it is worth noting that the desire for parental attention is also a factor which accounts for many non-incestuous teenage pregnancies. First, many teenagers use sexual activity as a warning flag to attract parental concern. But many parents fail to see that the teenager's promiscuity is actually an appeal for greater parental involvement and even discipline. So instead the parents tolerate or even condone the sexual activity by simply telling the teen to "be careful." This response simply drives the daughter (or son) to strive for even more outrageous conduct. Frequently pregnancy is seen as the last taboo—it is one thing the parents can't ignore. So the daughter subconsciously seeks to become pregnant in order to finally arouse her parents and force them to see her life and be a part of it. (Maloof, 73) The victim of incest, also seeking a true parental care and concern, thinks and acts similarly.

6. Ibid., 84.

7. Mary Jean Doe, "Incest and the Abortion Clinic," *The American Feminist*, Vol. 4 (4), Winter 1997-98, 15-16.

8. Maloof, "The Consequences of Incest," 89.

9. Ibid., 81.

10. Mecklenburg, *Abortion and Social Justice*, eds., Thomas W. Hilgers and Dennis J. Horan (New York: Sheed and Ward, 1972), 50.

11. Maloof, "The Consequences of Incest," 82 and 99.

12. Ibid., 99-101.

13. David C. Reardon, *Aborted Women, Silent No More*, (Chicago: Loyola University Press, 1987), 217-218.

CHAPTER EIGHT

TESTIMONIES OF INCEST VICTIMS WHO HAD ABORTIONS

"All I think of is, 'I should have done more, fought more, struggled more for the life of my child.'"
—"Denise Kalasky"

Forced to have sex with her father, Denise became pregnant. When the pregnancy was discovered, she refused to have an abortion. However, her father found an abortionist who performed the abortion without her consent.

I was a victim of incest, one of the "hard cases" for abortion. I was raped by my father when I was fifteen years old. It was not the first time, nor would it be the last. However, this time, I became pregnant.

One night, I became very sick and my parents took me to the hospital. I believe now that they knew I was pregnant since they took me to a different hospital than normal. The emergency room doctor discovered that, along with a very bad case of the flu, I was 19 weeks pregnant.

My father flew into a rage, accusing me of all sorts of things, and demanding I have an abortion. The doctor informed me that I was pregnant and asked me what I wanted. I had seen the "Silent Scream" in high school religion class and knew that abortion was murder. In spite of the pain and guilt I felt, knowing who the father of the baby was, it was far better to have a baby than the alternative—to kill it. I refused to have an abortion.

My father flew into an uncontrollable rage and demanded that I consent to the abortion, or that the doctor do it with or without my permission. The doctor refused because of my wishes. My father demanded that an abortionist be found—regardless of the cost.

Within one hour, this man arrived at the hospital, talked with my parents and decided to do the abortion, without speaking to me. I refused and tried to get off the examining table. He then asked three nurses to hold me while he strapped me to the bed and injected me with a muscle relaxant to keep me from struggling while he prepared to kill my baby. I continued to scream that I didn't want an abortion. He told me, "Shut up and quit that yelling!" Eventually, I was placed under general anesthesia and my child was brutally killed.

I was told that an abortion would solve my problem, when it was never really the problem in the first place.

I was told, "Your parents know what's best," when they obviously were only concerned about their own reputations.

I was told, "You made the right decision," when I was never given a choice. More important, where was my baby's choice?

I grieve every day for my daughter. I have struggled to forget the abuse and the abortion. I can do neither. All I think of is, "I should have done more, fought more, struggled more for the life of my child."

My situation may not be common, but I know it's not unique either. The emotions and problems I've had to deal with as a result of my abortion *are* common. The trauma of the rape and abuse were only intensified by the abortion. The guilt of knowing my baby is dead is something I will have to live with for the rest of my life.

I was violated and betrayed over and over by my father, who God created to love and protect me. I was humiliated, hurt, and violated again by the abortionist.

Why do even pro-lifers talk about making exceptions for abortion in cases of rape and incest, as if that is a way to have "compassion" for the mother? Why is this the only "loving" response to the situation? I have talked with "pro-lifers" who consider my abortion acceptable, under the circumstances. I want to tell people, *"If you really want to be compassionate, give this mother the opportunity to choose life for her child. If you really love the mothers who have been victimized, don't let them be exploited again by someone who will make a profit from their dead child — a memory that will haunt them for the rest of their lives."*

The next time you hear of the "hard cases," please remind people that every crisis pregnancy is difficult for the mother. If you believe these cases are hard, you're correct—they are extremely hard for the mother. But if you choose abortion, it's an *impossible* situation for the baby. The mom needs love, support and understanding, not the pain of allowing herself to be violated again in order to kill her child. Regardless of the circumstances, regardless of the pain involved, that helpless, innocent child has no voice, no defense, and no chance, unless we offer real love and real compassion to the mother.

My abortion was over five years ago. God is still healing me, but it has been a difficult fight. I hesitated to write to you because, although I'm actively pro-life, very few people know my story. It's still very difficult to share with people; however, I wanted to encourage you in your uncompromising stand for life.

"He heals the brokenhearted and binds up their wounds." (Psalm 147:3) God bless you!

"Often I cry. Cry because I could not stop the attacks. Cry because my daughter is dead. And I cry because it still hurts."
— Edith Young

When Edith was twelve, she became pregnant as the result of rape/incest by her stepfather. To cover up the incident, her parents procured an abortion for her without telling her what was to happen. The emotional and physical scars of her incest and abortion experiences are still with her today. This testimony was written in 1986 when Edith was 37 years old.

Where do I begin? Rape/incest and abortion. For most people, these things will never happen to them or anyone they know. When reported in the media, rape/incest is usually called by the watered-down term of child molestation or sexual abuse. By any name, it's still a tragedy. Abortion, though legal, is also a tragedy. Both take away from the victim things that cannot be replaced.

My remembrances of most of the occurrences are very vivid, even though they happened 26 years ago. These events began in 1960, and their effects continue still in 1986.

When I was 11 years old, I began my menstrual period. Shortly afterwards, I became the victim of rape/incest. Rape because it was violent and by force. Incest because the perpetrator was my stepfather, who by marrying my mother had assumed the position of my father.

Several times before the attacks, my stepfather entered my room and laid on the floor beside my bed. In the beginning, he didn't touch me or say anything to me. He'd pretend to be asleep, but I knew he wasn't. My mother, who was home during these times, would come to my room and make him leave. All she ever said to him was, "Leroy, get up and come out of here." She didn't say anything to me. She'd just leave, too.

One night she didn't leave as usual. Instead, she lifted my covers, opened my legs and asked if he had messed with me. I told her no. I began to be afraid, after this. Questions started going through my head: Messed with me how? What was he supposed to do to me that made her look between my legs? Oh God, help me, what's going on?

Not knowing what to expect, I started getting my two younger nieces to sleep with me. I felt safe with one on each side. But mom stopped them from sleeping with me immediately, while my stepfather continued to enter my room. Often I have felt that I was set up for all that was to happen to me—so conveniently being left alone with no assurance of protection.

Frequently, while mom was working, I was left alone with him. My sister and brother would be out, unaware of what was happening. They were both older than me, my sister by ten years and my brother by two. I also have a brother who was about five at this time. I can't remember much about him except I resented him. He is the only child my mother and stepfather had together.

Although there were several attacks, the one I remember most vividly is the first one. There was no one home but us. Maybe my younger brother was in bed, and I had also gone to bed. My stepfather entered my room the same as before, except this time he did not lay on the floor but started to climb onto my bed. I was terrified. I didn't know what he was going to do, but I knew I had to get away.

In the struggle, I knocked over a table lamp. He grabbed my leg, pulled me back onto the bed, yanked my clothes off, then he began to sexually attack me. I recall screaming, "No! No! Get away! Leave me alone! Someone help me!"

But it was all to no avail. There was no one to help me, no one to rescue me. So he continued, obviously sure he had time to do what he wanted, with no fear of being caught. This attack continued for what seemed to be forever. I was wondering to myself, "How could he do this to me? How could he be enjoying this? It hurts so bad. Why doesn't somebody help me? Why don't I die? Help! Help! Help!"

When he stopped, he threatened to hurt me and the rest of my family, including my natural father. He walked out as if what had happened was so natural. It meant nothing to him. But it meant something to me. I was left alone, crying softly so no one would hear me. I was so scared. I didn't move for a long time.

Mom came home, checking me as usual. I could tell from the look on her face that she knew. After all, I was bleeding. Nevertheless, she said nothing. She didn't even ask the usual, "Did he mess with you?" Instead, she left my room and got into bed with him. That was the last night she checked me.

From that night on, terror reigned in my life. I was being sexually abused, threatened by him, and betrayed by mom's silence. Even though she knew, I was still left alone with him; therefore the attacks continued. In the midst of these attacks, I tried to deny what was happening to me. But I have learned that denial is temporary, reality is forever.

I told no one about what was happening. Who could I tell? Mom and he were considered upstanding members of the community and church. People were always commenting on what a wonderful job they were doing in raising us. Several times I wanted to shout the truth, especially when I had been attacked the day before. But fear kept me from saying anything. What if I told and no one believed me? I would have to go home with them. Would he make good on his threats? What would mom do? She hadn't stopped him. I believed silence on my part was both my protector and friend.

One night, in January of 1961, mom and I walked to the doctor's office not far from where we lived. I didn't know why we were going. He was an elderly man with a kind face. He examined me and told mom I was about three or four months pregnant. I knew being pregnant meant having a baby, but I said nothing until the doctor asked me, "Who did this?" I replied, "My stepfather."

Of course, mom denied the truth. She said, "It was some old boy she's been messing with." Her answer was so strange to me. I was only twelve years old. I had better not look at a boy, let alone have one for a boyfriend. I didn't have any desire for one; the thought terrified me. We left his office and went home.

Within a couple of days, mom started giving me some large red pills. I didn't know where she got them, but I took them for a few days. Every day she would ask if I had started bleeding. She didn't explain anything, she just kept asking over and over if I was bleeding. Suddenly, I realized I was no longer being attacked sexually. Relief didn't come, though. There was a constant fear it would start again.

When the pills didn't bring about any bleeding, I was taken to another doctor. As we entered the office, I noticed no one was there but us. He led me to the examining table. I was too scared to talk. He said things such as "Hi, how are you?" and "It won't take long."

As I laid there, I looked around, asking myself, "What won't take long?" It was an ordinary doctor's office; he saw patients every day. My eyes wandered toward the foot of the table. I saw a red rubber tube in his hand. This was inserted into my vagina, there was a tug, then the tube was removed. I got off the table and joined my mother in the other room. We went home.

I had to stay in her room, in *their* bed. Again she began to ask if I felt or saw anything. I was told to use the basin whenever I felt "something" coming. I was alone when I began to feel "something." I got the basin and out "something" came.

The "something" was a baby girl. Yes, "something" was unquestionably a girl—my daughter. I saw her with my eyes, after she came from inside my body, lying there dead, in a cold white basin. What happened to her? I don't know, but I'll never forget her. She had a face, hands, arms, legs, and a body. Everything I had, she had. After seeing my baby, I don't remember what happened. Did I scream, call my mother, or what? I really don't remember.

Mom came in the room, and told me to lay down while she got me some bath water. She bathed me in the tub as if I had become as helpless as the baby in the basin. Maybe for the moment I was. Almost with every stroke, she made me a promise—promises she has never kept. For a while, I believed things would get better if she would just keep her promises. I believed the confusion, fear, and pain would disappear. However, all the stroking and promises in the world could not erase what I had experienced. It was like being in a dream world where all the dreams are nightmares. I thought I would awaken and find the nightmare was over. But it was not a dream, and the nightmare continues . . .

There weren't any more sexual assaults, but my mother started beating me for anything and everything. It seemed as if my mere existence was excuse enough. Mothers are supposed to love and protect, not betray and destroy.

It was when I was in the tenth grade taking nursing courses that I began to fully realize what happened to me. Imagine the shock when I understood what took place that day. The day I passed "something"—my baby, my daughter Lori Ann—into a basin. My textbook said that "life begins at conception." Reality really sunk in. A life had ended that day. Murder had been committed.

After this revelation, I started drinking. Liquor was easy to get. My stepfather drank all the time, so I began stealing his hidden alcohol. I did not worry about being caught. In fact, I didn't care.

Alcohol helped me through the next few years. Drinking made existing easier; it distorted reality enough to go on while truthfully my life was in a turmoil. Yet no one knew it. I was an honor roll student. In fact, I was on the National Honor Society in high school. From the sixth to twelfth grade I sang in the school choir. In high school, I participated in intramural sports and was the captain of the girl's basketball team.

They stayed together approximately 12 or 13 years after the abortion. How she could continue to stay with him, I'll never understand . . . I tried to kill him a few times. Once by making him move when his nose was hemorrhaging, by throwing something out of his reach. Three times I attempted to stab him, but mom intervened each time. How I hated her for that. During those attempts I was upset by my failure to kill him. Now, I'm grateful to God that I didn't succeed. Living with the memory of sexual attacks, pregnancy, abortion, and beatings are more than enough without adding murder.

When I was a senior in high school mom decided she didn't want me around anymore. I moved in with my natural father. You may have been wondering where he was during this time. He and mom separated and divorced when I was about three or four years old. I saw him often, though. Since he was included in the threats of my stepfather, I did not tell him about the attacks. I had vowed to never tell him. All I kept thinking was: What would he do? Would he be killed like my baby? Would it kill him to know? Would he kill them and end up in jail?

I was so afraid to tell him, and only did so in September 1986 when I was serving as the Delaware State Director for Women Exploited by Abortion, a post-abortion support group. A press conference was to be held and I didn't want him to read about me or hear it from someone else. He was 77 years old.

Telling daddy was one of the hardest things I have ever had to do. God's timing was perfect. Our national president, Lorijo

Nerad, was there to support me. Daddy wept when he was alone but he said he was sorry, he didn't know.

The Lord has blessed me with three living children. I became pregnant before I moved out of my mother's, while I was a senior in high school. The school's answer was adoption. Arrangements were made without my knowledge or consent. Refusal was made in not so polite terms by me.

The pregnancy was not too bad. I carried my son full term. Ironically, one of my daughters was born on January 22, 1973, the day abortion was legalized.

Throughout the years I have been depressed, suicidal, furious, outraged, lonely, and have felt a sense of loss. I have felt, and at times still feel, that my mother and stepfather owe me something. What? I don't know. Maybe a sincere, "I'm sorry."

Even if my daughter had been put up for adoption, instead of killed, some of the pain would not be present. Often I cry. Cry because I could not stop the attacks. Cry because my daughter is dead. And I cry because it still hurts. They say time heals all wounds. This is true. But it doesn't heal the memories, at least not for me.

I've suffered many physical problems and continue to do so. Ever since the abortion, I've suffered chronic infections of my tubes, ovaries and bladder. The pains from my menstrual periods were nightmarish and continued from the time of my abortion until my partial hysterectomy in November 1982. In April of this year, I again had surgery. There was a growing, bleeding cyst on my left ovary. On my right side, there was a massive amount of adhesions and the ovary could not be found. Twenty-five years have gone by but the consequences of the abortion are still going on.

As you can see, the abortion which was to be "in my best interest" just has not been. As far as I can tell, it only "saved their reputations," "solved their problems," and allowed their lives to go merrily on.

My daughter, how I miss her so. I miss her regardless of the reason for her conception. You see, she was a part of me, an innocent human being, sentenced to death because of the selfish, sexual gratification of another and the need to "save reputations." She was a unique individual whose life was exterminated.

Yes, the abortion occurred before the ill-fated legalization of abortion in 1973. Not in a back alley, but in a sterile office, on the examining table of a doctor, much like the abortion mills of today. Everyone is still living except for my daughter and both doctors.

In situations like mine, emotions are something you are expected to control no matter what. I wasn't allowed to cry, scream, react, or grieve. These things are also true of women who have abortions today. Whatever the reason, a baby is killed and his or her mother is left to face the reality of that decision, often alone.

In the past, incest was not spoken of. Like abortion, it was taboo in our country. But a few years ago when incest stories became a common headline for reporters, I wondered what was happening psychologically to the many women who have been victims of incest. What changes were they going through? Now I wonder what's going to happen to the millions of women who have had abortions when reporters finally get the guts to write as honestly about abortion as they did about incest. All the legalities in the world will not remove the reality that a baby is a baby. For many women the aborted baby is the only one they ever had a chance to have. For many more, abortion is the start of physical and/or emotional complications.

The attacks, the abortion, and my baby in the basin frequently return in my dreams. There have been a countless number of nights when I've gone without sleep just so I wouldn't dream. I still have these sleepless nights, not for me, but for the millions of babies who are still dying. I lose sleep whenever I picket or sidewalk counsel at an abortuary. Watching woman after woman go in hurts. I know that the solution to their situations will not be found in there. Problems are not ended by abortion, but only made worse.

Even though I didn't have any say about the abortion, it has had a greater impact on my life than the rape/incest. About nine years ago, I accepted Christ as my personal Savior. He has since become not only my Savior, but also Lord of my life. I have repented of the sin of abortion because of my years of silence. I am free.

It's because of Christ I am able to tell my story. It's not easy, but I pray that by telling it an abused person seeks help, a baby is saved, and most importantly, a woman who is considering abortion will save herself.

Reprinted with permission from Aborted Women, Silent No More *by David*

"How did abortion affect me? It is not unlike living with sexual abuse . . . I weep for the life I could have saved. The pain will be there all my life."
                                                              —"Ellen Carson"

Ellen became pregnant at 14 after being conditioned to have sex with a family member. Convinced by the perpetrator that the baby would have medical problems because of the incest, she lied about her age and had an abortion. Many years later, she still struggles with the hurt brought on by her abortion.

At the age of 14, I had a secret. I was not only sexually active, but had been conditioned to have sex with a member of my family. At times, this secret pulled me into depression. However, I was able to hide my abuse from others, as well as myself. I craved love and affection. I was confused by my blossoming sexuality. And I was unhappy about what was expected of me. But the summer of 1979 shattered my emotions.

It had been several months since my last period. I never paid much attention, as part of my denial that something bad was happening to me. But suddenly I realized I was pregnant. The idea of having a baby seemed unreal to me, but I found myself excited at the prospect. I longed for the pure and selfless love a mother and child can share. Yet I was worried that becoming pregnant by a family member would create deformities that could be dangerous to me and a child.

I soon told my abuser of the suspicion, and he agreed it had been three or four months since my last period. He confirmed my fears of a "monster baby" and wiped my tears. He convinced me that abortion was the only alternative I had. He handed me the money and sent me on my way.

Three days later I sat in a clinic in Seattle. I signed papers relieving them of any responsibility, should something go wrong. I gave a false name, address, birth date and number of weeks pregnant. I looked much younger than my 14 years, but no one seemed concerned. This was "minor surgery." I wanted comfort, but no one knew about my life . . .

I allowed the nurse to sedate me, and the procedure began on schedule. Many hours later I stared into space, and wished I didn't feel so empty. Someone said I had been at least 22 weeks pregnant . . . I wanted to feel the life inside me, but it could never return.

I am no longer a victim, but a survivor. I struggle with the guilt and pain of my abortion. My family consoles me with reasons why it was all right that I had an abortion, but my mother and sister are as hurt as I.

I had hoped someone would question me before my abortion. But I was not asked to prove my age or identity. I was never asked why I chose abortion. If I had been questioned at all, someone would have heard quite a story . . . I feel the state let me down.

If abortion had been questioned in my case, I may have had a baby. I may have been happier. I may not have gone through the suicide attempts. I know that abortion has long term affects on women . . . I have no doubt that other young girls have been through abortions for reasons like me . . .

How did abortion affect me? It is not unlike living with sexual abuse. I fear I have been guilty of a misdeed. I weep for the life I could have saved. The pain will be there all my life.

I hope other young girls will learn from my mistake.

Previously published as part of a collection of letters in "About my abortion: Women write to tell of personal experiences," The Daily News, Longview, Wash., April 11, 1990, p. C2.

"The memories of the abortion itself are horrible, but even more painful is the fact that I killed a child . . . I have often wondered what my child would be like today if I hadn't had an abortion."

—"Carla Harris"

"Carla's" stepfather began sexual abusing her when she was 13. When she became pregnant two years later, he told her that abortion was her only option. Carla did as she was told, but could not shake the pain of the experience. Even though she now has a young son to love, she is haunted by the memory of the child she lost to abortion.

When I was about 13, my stepfather started molesting me. It continued until I came forward with it when I was 16. At age 15, I became pregnant. No one knew but my stepfather and a lady that told him where to take me.

My stepfather told me the only way was to have an abortion. He made me set up an appointment; he dropped me off and picked me up.

I could not tell anyone what had happened. I was messed up after this. I couldn't take much more, so I finally told what was happening to me. On top of all my other problems, the biggest emotional hurt was the killing of that child. I have often wondered what my child would be like today, if I hadn't had an abortion.

I am pretty much over the effects of the molestation, but I still have to face a lot of effects from the abortion. The memories of the abortion itself are horrible, but even more painful is the fact that I killed a child. I wonder if it was a boy or a girl, what color hair it had, and all of the other things a parent sees.

I am happily married now and have been for three years. My husband and I have been blessed with a little boy who is one now. I am thankful that the Lord protected me, so I could have the blessing of giving birth.

Thank you for showing the public the truth of the abortion issue. I have always said that I wish the pro-choicers could see it through my eyes.

"One week after the abortion [my sister] took her life . . . Her three children are growing up without their mom because no one wanted to ask questions."
—"Julie Anderson"

"Julie" and her sister were both victims of incest. Although Julie never became pregnant from the incest, her sister did—and had an abortion at age 16. Following a second abortion years later, her sister committed suicide. Julie believes that had anyone questioned her sister before the abortions and tried to meet her real needs, her sister might be alive today.

My sister and I were both victims of incest. My sister was being sexually assaulted by my brothers for a number of years when she got her first abortion at the age of sixteen. Had she been questioned by anyone as to how a minor like herself had come to be pregnant in the first place, perhaps she could have been saved from any further abuse within the family.

This is indeed what should have happened in any agency that claims to be concerned about preventing child abuse. As it turned out, she was given the abortion without my parents' consent or knowledge and then returned to the same environment.

Years later, after having given birth to three children, and having had many years of psychotherapy and antidepressant drugs, she became pregnant in a crisis situation. She was advised by friends and self-appointed do-gooders to abort the baby to take care of herself. This caused her a great deal of distress and anxiety. The decision was very difficult for her and in her weakened state she succumbed to the "sensibility" of their arguments and scheduled the abortion.

She was crying when she entered the clinic, she cried throughout the procedure, and was sobbing as she left. No one at the clinic asked her any questions that might upset her any more. But of course, had anyone asked her, they might have recognized that she was not emotionally strong enough to stand the abortion. Had they inquired about her health history they may have seen her as the high risk patient she was.

None of this took place. One week after the abortion she took her life with a gunshot to the chest, striking her heart. Her three children are growing up without their mom because no one wanted to ask questions.

I am suggesting nothing that would bar any healthy, determined woman from obtaining an abortion she is sure she wants. But abortion without regulation doesn't give her a chance to make all the decisions based on the true facts and the security of knowing that as much as possible has been done to protect her against criminal-minded persons and inferior medical practices.

Excerpted from Forbidden Grief: The Unspoken Pain of Abortion *by Theresa Karminski Burke with David C. Reardon (Springfield, IL: Acorn Books) scheduled for publication in Summer 2000.*

CHAPTER NINE

TESTIMONIES OF INCEST VICTIMS WHO GAVE BIRTH TO THEIR CHILDREN

"After my daughter was born, it was love at first sight . . . I know I made the right decision in having her."
—Nancy "Cole"

Nancy was molested by her father as child, and again as a teenager. When she became pregnant, her father manipulated her into telling everyone she didn't know who the child's father was. Although she suffered from the effects of the abuse for many years, she says her daughter gave her "a purpose and a reason to live."

From birth to age two-and-a-half, I lived with my natural mother and father. Although I have no memory of this period of time, a variety of sources from both sides of the family agree on what took place. My parents argued frequently, my father battered my mother, and they separated frequently.

My dad was 22 and my mom 15 when they married. They had three children in the next five years: a boy, a girl (me), then another boy. My parents were separated at the time of my mother's death. My father killed my mother, stating, "If I can't have my family, no one else is going to."

My father was incarcerated for this from the time I was two until I was seven. My brothers and I lived with my father's aunt and uncle during this time.

My father began molesting me when I was seven, telling me that he was "teaching me." He would arrange opportunities for us to be alone so he could take advantage of me.

I wasn't sure whether what was happening was normal or not. My dad presented the situation to me as if everyone did the same, yet my aunt and uncle were raising me and teaching me to be modest, almost to an extreme. But since I had never had a dad before, I couldn't be sure.

I didn't enjoy what I was experiencing; I was mentally

repulsed by it and physically hurt. An extra dimension was that my dad would tell my brothers that he was taking me in the bedroom to punish me for being bad. But I did like the attention that my dad gave me; no one had ever really treated me special prior to that.

I finally told a friend about what was happening and she told her mother, who told my aunt. I came home from school one day and my aunt asked me about it. She took me on her lap and coaxed the information out of me. It took several hours as I was reluctant to tell her. My dad had told me not to tell, but I don't remember any threats being made at this time. When my uncle came home from work, he asked me if I was telling the truth and I said yes.

I didn't hear anymore about it for several days. My aunt kept me home from school but didn't say why. I was upset about missing school and didn't understand what was going on. My aunt finally told me in the car (en route) that we were going to the doctor. She told me we were going to get me checked to see if I had worms. There was no mention or connection made to what had occurred with my dad.

My aunt reported the molestation to the police. Two police officers came out to my school. I was summoned to the principal's office where they were waiting to transport me downtown to the police station.

At the police station, I was questioned by a woman about what had happened. But she used anatomical terms and I didn't understand them. So I answered many of her questions with "I don't know." I was frightened and intimidated. The woman told me, "We can't help you if you don't answer the questions." Help me with what, I wondered. No explanations were given me at this time.

Some time later, my father was brought to trial on charges of incest. He was convicted, and I was told by my aunt, "It's over now; just forget it," and that was that. Or so I thought.

About a year-and-a-half or so later, I was told that my father had won a retrial. By the time of the retrial my memories of the molestation were somewhat blurred. I had been told to "forget it," and to some degree I had. Also, since I was older, many of the attorney's questions were embarrassing to me—too embarrassing to even answer.

As I walked down from giving my testimony, I stopped by the table where my dad sat with his attorney and said to him, "I'm sorry, Daddy." Even though throughout the court case my dad did everything in his power to prove that I was lying—that in fact I was a chronic liar—I still felt that I had betrayed him by telling.

My father was acquitted at this trial. But after that time (I think I was about nine years old) he stayed away from me until I was 14. When I was 15, my older brother graduated from high school. Having not seen my dad for five years or so, and not knowing why (no one had told my brothers about the molestation or the trials), my brother decided to look my dad up. This opened up a whole new can of worms.

My dad decided that he wanted to resume visitation with his children. My aunt and uncle said no at first, but when my dad threatened a court case, they told him just to completely take us. I was away at summer camp when this took place, and when I returned, all my things were packed. I moved in with my dad the next day.

Within a week my dad was sexually abusing me. It started with me asking him, "Did it (the prior abuse) really happen or did I make it up?" He responded by molesting me.

This time there was no one around to help. My father had encouraged me to cut off all ties with the family that had raised me. I was pregnant within four months of this time. My father had remarried and had me tell his wife that I didn't know who the father of the baby was, although my stepmother did suspect because I didn't even date.

I didn't tell anyone about the molestation. As I stated earlier, my dad had pretty much brainwashed me to do whatever he wanted. So I told everyone that I didn't know who the father was (which made me feel like a real low-life.)

When I first found out I was pregnant, at about four months, I was in denial. I was either sleeping or vomiting all the time, so I remained pretty numb to the reality of the whole thing. I was quite depressed and continued to have nausea and vomiting throughout the pregnancy.

I remained pretty much in denial or in a fantasy world throughout the pregnancy. I looked forward to having the baby in a fairy-tale sort of way. I thought she would be cute and cuddly—a doll to play with. I had played with dolls until I was fourteen, and I was only fifteen now. I thought she could be someone to love me.

I saw a set of obstetricians who saw me on alternating visits.

One was very pushy about me having an abortion, even up to the last month of my pregnancy. But my dad had let me know that it was not an option, and I was obedient. I don't know what I wanted.

After my daughter was born, it was love at first sight. She gave me a reason to live and a sense of purpose. But I suffered from the effects of the abuse for many years until I became a Christian five years ago. The Lord healed me of many years of deep depression.

I know I made the right decision in having my daughter. I believe emphatically that abortion is murder and should never be an option. The other two options—adoption or raising the child—should be decided on a totally individual basis, considering the best interests of both the mother and the child.

In the case of rape or incest, abortion is an attempt to erase what cannot be healed. It transforms the victim into a perpetrator; she was a victim of sexual abuse, but now she becomes a murderer.

Women who become pregnant as a result of incest are frequently told that their baby will be a monster or that their child will be stigmatized and never have a normal life or be happy. They are often manipulated into having abortions by this fear. But my daughter is now 18, loves the Lord, and is happy and well adjusted. I have raised her all her life and I know I made the right decision.

I do believe that counseling should be made available throughout the pregnancy and as long afterwards as is necessary or desirable by the mother—even if it is a number of years. To women who are in situations similar to mine, we need to be instruments of the Lord's love and healing. I would offer the love of God to them and point them to Him who is the Source of all healing and comfort.

"God is slowly healing all of our emotional scars . . . I have peace in my life now which only His presence can bring."
—"Linda March"

As a child, Linda was a victim of horrible physical, mental, and sexual abuse. Impregnated by her stepfather, she tried to abort the life growing inside her. But she says today that she is grateful that she allowed her son to live, and that God is healing the many wounds in her life.

My life has not been an easy one. It has been filled with the ramifications of the sins of others since my conception. My mother decided to seek revenge upon her husband for some minor offense via an adulterous affair with his best friend. I was the result of her "mistake." She was subsequently divorced and my biological father left her to face the consequences of her affair alone.

We lived with my mom's parents, and my grandmother never missed the opportunity to remind her, and me, of the "sin and shame" we had brought into her life. My earliest memories are filled with the bitter arguments and strife between my mother and grandmother. The situation became so difficult to bear that my mother began to drink heavily and to have numerous affairs with men in order to escape the hellish situation in which she was forced to live.

We finally moved into a tiny two-bedroom apartment when my mother could no longer tolerate things at home. It was then that my own nightmare began in earnest.

My mother had become an alcoholic by this time and would sell herself, body and soul, to any man who would feed her addiction. She was looking for love in all the wrong places and when she could not find it, she vented that frustration on me, whom she imagined to be the source of all her problems.

Mother would disappear for days at a time, leaving a frightened seven-year-old home alone. There would be no food, no water, no power, and no phone in the house. I vividly remember roaming the streets in search of returnable drink bottles to sell to buy what little food I had.

I have horrible memories of terrible physical and mental abuse. Memories of being locked out of the apartment during the dead of winter, forced to sleep in the car without even a coat, so my mother could entertain her "guests." But soon she lost all sense of decency and I witnessed acts of depravity that no child should ever have to see. Senseless acts of violence which no human being should ever inflict on another.

All of this finally reached the point where I began to emulate the behavior to which I was constantly exposed. My grandparents stepped in and had me removed from my mother's custody. I was sent to live with my aunt and uncle in Florida. It was there that I learned what life in a normal Christian family was supposed to be. For the first time in my life, I was at peace.

During my stay in Florida, I was taught about Christ, and I think it was there that I accepted Him as my personal Savior. God intervened in my life before I was irrevocably ruined by Satan and his demons. My peace did not last long, however. Three years later, while I was visiting my grandparents while my aunt and uncle were on vacation, my mother reappeared. With her was the man who was to become my tormentor—her new husband, my stepfather.

After I was removed from my mother's custody, her world had fallen completely apart. Her boyfriend was confined to a mental institution for alcoholism. My mother lost her job, and consequently her home, her car, her personal possessions, and what was left of her dignity.

My stepfather literally picked her up out of the gutter in which she was living and married her. He spirited her away to Connecticut, and no one in the family knew her whereabouts until she suddenly reappeared on my grandparents' doorstep.

My first reaction to her husband was one of horror, for all those repressed, vivid memories of the past came flooding back into my mind. It was soon after this initial meeting that he began to show his true intentions toward me. They had rented an apartment and wanted me to come live with them. I had no intention of doing so, but despite everything that had happened in the past, I still loved my mother. My stepfather's threat of something dire happening to my mother if I refused worked quite well.

When my aunt and uncle returned for me, I reluctantly informed them of my decision to remain with my mother and her new husband. I had no desire to live with this man, but the threat was fresh in my mind. I really believed that he would have done something to my mother. It was then that my ordeal began at the age of eleven.

The next six years or so were filled with every kind of abuse known to mankind. Physical, mental, sexual, verbal—I experienced them all, to their fullest depraved extent. School became my refuge, and the Lord saw fit to give me a baby brother to love. He became the focal point of my existence, for if he had not come into my life at that critical period, I seriously do not believe that I could have survived my ordeal with even a tiny amount of sanity remaining.

All during this time, I prayed every night, sometimes until

dawn, for divine deliverance from hell. I frequently went to bed with a knife under my pillow, intent upon murder, and just as frequently, went to bed with thoughts of suicide.

I was 14 when I became pregnant. Abortion was not legal in 1968, but had abortion been an option at that time, my son would, in all probability, would not be here with me today. And I would have missed out on one of the few joys of my life. As it was, when I discovered I was pregnant with my son, I despised the tiny life which was growing in my womb, and tried to abort him. But God knew best, and allowed him to live.

My son was born a month before my fifteenth birthday. The decision was made for me by my mother that I would keep my son and raise him. She deemed that if "I was woman enough to have him, then I was woman enough to raise him."

I received my deliverance one day when I finally had quite enough of the abuse. That day had included a particularly violent display of his incestuous lust. It was the first time I ever fought back. I honestly believe he would have killed me if I had not shot at him with the very pistol he used to threaten me with so many times before. I went to the police and informed them of my plight. My stepfather was arrested for incest, crime against nature, and assault on a minor female. He was convicted of his crimes and spent the next 13 years in prison.

I spent the next 21 years of my life in a vain attempt to escape the bondage of my stepfather's sin. It was in 1990 that God began to gently remind me of His presence in my life, and believe me, I fought Him with every ounce of my being. For if I accepted God into my life, I could no longer live in the fantasy world I had created for myself in order to cope with all that had transpired before. I would have to face reality, and I did not want to do that.

As a result of my ordeal I became a loner, for I did not trust anyone. The only three people I allowed into my inner circle were my grandfather, my brother, and eventually, my son. I wrapped all the bitterness, rage, hatred, humiliation, guilt, self-loathing, shame, and distress into a tight little ball and suppressed it into the deepest recesses of my mind.

What my parents robbed me of can never be totally accounted for in this life. They robbed me of my childhood. They effectively robbed me of all of my hopes, plans, and dreams I had for the future. My stepfather's sick lust robbed my husband of my virtue and my son of a father. My son and I enjoy a close relationship now, but that was not always the case.

We are okay now, but it has been a very long struggle. I met and married a man whom I credit God for sending my way. I did not think it possible for me to love any man the way I love my husband. I still have many emotional scars, especially where sex is involved, but I pray my husband always has patience with me. I suffer from manic depression, which will require medication for the rest of my life. I have diabetes, which I have difficulty finding the self-discipline to control. I have a volatile temper, which I keep under rigid self-control. But with the help of God, and my husband, I am gradually becoming a whole person.

But one positive thing I have developed from all the chaos of my life is a deep-seated hatred for all that is sin. I am forever grateful to God for delivering me from the temptation to dabble in the things so many of those who have experienced my situation have turned to for solace. I still sin daily, but with the grace of God, I am learning.

The sinful legacy my stepfather left on everyone he touched is still quite evident today. God is slowly healing all of our emotional scars, but then, He never promised us a rose garden. I have peace in my life now which only His presence can bring.

"I wanted to keep my baby. I could not stand the thought of anything else."

—**"Dana Lewis"**

"Dana" was sexually abused by her father for six years. When she threatened to tell her mother, her father raped her and she became pregnant. She decided to keep her child and with her mother's love and support, made it through her pregnancy and gave birth to a son. Although she still has a long way to go in dealing with the pain of her abuse, she is comforted by the presence of her child.

I have tried to forget most of my past life, but I think it was pretty happy. I drew a lot; I wanted to be an artist. My personality was sort of withdrawn into myself; I'm very shy. My family life was not. My father ran around on my mother. (I hated my father for doing this to her.) They yelled back and forth some, but not a lot.

I was 14 years old when my father first started to do these

things to me. At first I felt a lot of guilt. I thought it was my fault, but I have since learned that it was not my fault. He is very sick.

When I was 20 years old I told him to stop, that I had enough and I was going to tell mom. He said that I had better not and left. But then he came back. He had been drinking, and he told me that I had better never talk, and then he raped me.

I was very angry and am still very upset. My mother and my brother are the only ones (other than my father) who know about this. My brother did not talk about it. He is only my half-brother, but he was very close to me at this time. My mom does not talk much about it because I do not want to talk about it. I sensed love and understanding from my mom and brother for me, but I know they are very angry toward my father.

I was five months pregnant before I went to the doctor. I about died when I learned I was pregnant. I never once hated the baby, but I just didn't know what to think.

I wanted to keep my baby. I could not stand the thought of anything else. As the pregnancy progressed I felt that well, I am going to be a mother and this is my child. The hardest thing to deal with was becoming a mother one year after graduation. Life had just begun for me. But the best thing was that I had my mother there to help me.

After my mom got over the shock of it being my father's baby she was very happy, yet sick at the same time. She was very helpful and understanding and she helped me very much. My mother and brother's feelings for me are probably the only things that kept me from blowing my brains away.

The rest of my family was upset because I was having this baby and was not married. Like I said, they did not know, and they still don't know about the sexual abuse but "Ryan" looks so much like my father that I'm sure they have guessed. After I had Ryan, they treated me like nothing was wrong, but they sort of held me at arm's length.

After this happened I pushed it all away; I pushed all feelings about the rape away. I don't talk about it, and I don't think about it. Before all this incest happened I loved my father but blamed him for his and mother's problems. Now I hate the man. I don't care if I have anything to do with another man again.

Ryan is four-and-a-half-years old, and I am not sure how or when I will tell him about his birth. I definitely think children in this situation are discriminated against. People who do not understand, people who have never had this happen to their family, look down on you as someone very low. Children who are born of incest are looked down upon . . . people think they are probably retarded because of the incest.

If someone had asked me about three-and-a-half years ago if having my baby would improve my life in any way, I would have said no. But Ryan has kept me from doing a lot of dumb things. I don't think women should get an abortion even if the child will be retarded. They are human; they are real people. They aren't things we can throw away when one looks like it won't be "right." If the woman for some reason or another cannot keep her child—if she can't support it or if she's just a baby herself—I think adoption is great.

By rights, I of all people should have had an abortion because I was having my own father's baby. But I did not and I thank the Lord I did not. Ryan is very intelligent. He is fine and there is nothing wrong with him.

To a woman who is in a similar situation I would say that I know what she is going through, and there are people who care. I would tell her to quit blaming herself because it is not her fault.

CHAPTER TEN

TESTIMONIES OF CHILDREN CONCEIVED IN INCEST

"God planned for us to be here, and may use us for His glory through our situation."

—**"Sara Judge"**

"Sara" is the daughter of Nancy "Cole," whose testimony as an incest survivor was in the previous chapter. She was raised by her mother and says she is "living proof" that children conceived in these situations can live a happy life.

My mother was a victim of sexual abuse. The sexual assaults began when she was around seven. Prior to that, she was living with her aunt and uncle. Her father was doing time in jail for her mother's murder. He killed her in a pre-meditated car accident.

Her father brainwashed her into thinking that it was her fault that the car crashed, killing her mother. He convinced her that it was perfectly normal to have a sexual relationship together.

I don't remember how I found out about the incest. I feel as if I have always known. At first, I was bothered to find out that I was an incest baby. But now I have just faced this knowledge as a fact I will always have to deal with. I have accepted it and am not angry or guilt-ridden.

I have no hatred towards my biological father, nor towards my mother. Without them, I might not be here today. Without the cleansing of the blood of Christ, I would be an emotional wreck, and anger-filled toward life. I am happy and have accepted my background. I would even like to have children of my own some day.

Recently, I wrote a letter to a newspaper columnist who printed letters that discussed incest. The general opinion was that a girl who conceives a child through incest was better off having an abortion. The readers agreed that the baby would be born retarded, but I am living proof that those opinions are false and cannot be proven true.

I feel abortion is wrong in all situations. The baby is innocent and doesn't deserve death because of its parentage. There are many loving people out there who would love to adopt a baby. I also believe there is nothing wrong with keeping the baby, either. After all, my mother kept me and is continuing to raise me.

Abortion is wrong. God planned for us to be here, and may use us for His glory through our situation.

"My mother sacrificed her needs for mine, carried a shame that wasn't hers, and brought a baby into this world that in this day and age probably would not have made it."
—"John Kent"

John feels extremely blessed by his natural mother's love and defense of his life, and the love he received from his adoptive parents. He is happy to have renewed his relationship with his natural mother.

I am as pro-life as you can get. I have a good reason to be. I'm alive.

I am the product of rape, and not only rape, but of incest. My mother sacrificed her needs for mine, carried a shame that wasn't hers, and brought a baby into this world that in this day and age probably would not have made it.

But she didn't stop there.

Being unable to provide me with the things a child needs—like security, food, a roof over my head, schooling—she denied herself the right to keep me, her child. She selflessly let me go for adoption when I was seven.

But my blessings didn't stop there, because many seven-year-olds don't get adopted. I was adopted in nine months by wonderful, spirit-filled parents who showed me Jesus, provided for me materially, and gave themselves unselfishly for my behalf.

Ten to eleven years later, Jesus brought my mom and I back together for our mutual healing. He healed us both.

Right now, I am almost twenty. I have a whole life ahead of me bound to be filled with jobs, work, a wife and children, Christmases, hobbies, vacations, sports, dreams, hopes, successes and failures, and two sets of parents whom I love more than I thought possible.

Mom, thank you for letting me live.

Mam, thank you for loving me boundlessly.
I love you both.

"Uniquely woman, uniquely me. That's what God made me to be."

—Dixie Lee Gourley

At the time she wrote this testimony, Dixie Lee was a 51-year-old nurse. As a child, she was placed in boarding homes where she was visited by her father who subjected her to incestuous abuse. It wasn't until she was 40 years old that she learned that he had also abused a little-known "half-sister" who was her real mother. Dixie Lee is proud of her mother, and happy to have a relationship with her and her family. Dixie Lee's faith and optimism, despite all the pain that she has suffered, is truly inspiring.

This is my personal testimony as one who was conceived by incest, and was later a victim of incest.

My mother grew up in a family that included her mother, father, and four brothers. She was the only female child.

While living at home, she experienced incest at the hands of her father that resulted in a pregnancy at 15 years of age. As her pregnancy progressed, she was exposed to procedures to hopefully get rid of me in the womb; to abort me! She still bears some effects of that abuse today.

All the procedures failed. God Almighty blocked man's plans. God had his plans and purposes for my life. I'm a "real" miracle. From the moment I was conceived, God's protective hand was on my life, and he was working out his purpose for this life.

I was born August 10, 1938, in a home for unwed mothers in Denver, Colorado. After my birth, my mother was sent out of state to stay with relatives to hide the shamefulness of my father.

From the time of my birth to 17 years of age, I never lived with my natural family. Through the Christian nurse that attended my mother at the time of my birth, contacts came from three of the five families I was later placed in.

I wasn't a foster child, nor was I adopted. I was a boarder. The first two families and the last family I grew up in were Christian families from the same Baptist church in Denver. The last family I resided in from about five years of age to early adulthood.

The families I was placed in knew the circumstances of my birth, but the amazing thing is, not once in all those years did they let it slip out to me.

Although placed in these different families, my natural father (who was also my "grandfather") would make weekly visits to see me and pay my room and board. When I was small, he often took me to the city park to see and feed the ducks. As I grew older, it would be a drive or ride, usually on a Saturday morning, or occasionally a planned picnic with "Mom G," my father's wife, who I grew up thinking was my mother. Occasionally we took a trip to the family mountain cabin. I never met any of the rest of the family during these years and there was never any mention of them.

God used the Christian families, their love and their lives, to influence me. The church was a big influence: Sunday School, Vacation Bible School, camps, club programs, etc. All were a big part of my life while growing up. I praise God for this. My experiences in life were varied, good experiences as well as unpleasant experiences. I had a normal life.

Unfortunately, even though I was staying with a Christian family, my natural father took advantage of me and I experienced incest over a period of six or seven years; from 11 to 16 years of age.

Sometimes on a Saturday morning my father would take me for a ride in the car to a secluded area along a country road. Other times, in the evening, he'd park in a dark area of town where he could carry out his actions in the front seat of the car. Occasionally, I experienced incest while at the family cabin. It was "our secret." He would usually give me some spending money after he completed his acts of incest.

This sexual abuse produced in me feelings of anger, guilt and hatred. I began to dread his visits. I was really relieved when he couldn't make his visits. If I had a choice to do something with the family I was living with, I preferred to be with them than with my father. He was affected by my choice in these cases, but he never made a big deal of it.

The family that I lived with at the time did not know of any of this abuse, although the mother occasionally appeared apprehensive after I returned from a visit with my father. When she would do my laundry and find a spot of grease on my underwear, she would question me as to how it got there. I would give an excuse to cover up the reason for the soiled underwear, but this made me feel uneasy, apprehensive, and depressed. There was some anger and fear at being questioned.

The negative feelings that I experienced as an incest victim lasted many years. It affected my desires for dating relationships. I did date a Christian fellow who was in the Air Force my senior year in high school. This was a friendship, no serious relationship. I did not date during college. The desire wasn't there. I feel that God had numbed my desires for marriage at this point in my life. I sense that he postponed my desire for a marriage relationship to allow time for *complete* healing of my experience as an incest victim.

For most of my adult life, I have lived alone, with the exception of college and nursing school. I've had a very interesting life. I have worked in the health field for 23 years, helping people in special times of their lives when they have been facing crisis experiences. Music has been a real vital part of my life. I enjoy reading, sewing, and embroidery. I have also been active as a club leader and camp counselor for "Pioneer Girls." I enjoy camping. I also enjoy keeping up correspondence with college friends and nursing classmates. This has resulted in some meaningful lifetime relationships.

In 1978, while I was working in a hospital in Vermont, I received a phone call from a relative of my natural family in California. "Mom G" was in the hospital facing some serious surgery and she requested that the family members to contact me and have me come to see her. She felt I could say something to her that would help her to face this crisis in her life. The family took care of all the travel arrangements for me.

When I arrived in California, I met two of my half-brothers (half-uncles?), and my "half-sister," who was actually my mother. I spent the next three weeks riding to the hospital with my "sister" and her husband.

Three days before I was to return to Vermont, another family member asked me, "Have you ever wondered who your real mother is?" I said no. I had never questioned that "Mom G" was my mother. So I met my natural family members, including my mother, at 40 years of age. It was a good experience because God had worked in a unique way on my life in the intervening years, preparing me for this special time in my life.

The knowledge of my background answered some observations I'd made in the earlier years as far as the coolness I'd felt when "Mom G" was in my presence. After I learned the truth, I felt she was hurting enough and that my questioning her would accomplish no positive effect, but only bring more pain.

I learned that at the time of my high school graduation, I had caused a stir in my natural family. An opportunity had developed that necessitated my needing a copy of my birth certificate. "Mom G" had made a trip to Idaho and had my natural mother sign papers so "Mom G" could adopt me. It was another layer in the cover up.

My life has been affected in a positive way by the discovery of my biological mother. I have added my natural family to the many other families that have had a special part in my life. Since meeting my natural family, I've been treated equally in family matters. My mother and stepdad have been so helpful to me, and have taken a real interest in my life. I feel very much a part of the family, and very grateful for having them in my life.

When I was ten years of age, the last time my mother remembered seeing me, she married a widower with two small boys. She never had any other children. I would like to get closer to my mother and stepdad, but there seems to still be some reservations. They're not open to discussing their true feelings.

I love my birth mother for giving me life. My life has touched so many other lives over these 51 years. I respect her for what she went through. I feel her hurt with her; and I've suggested that anytime she would want to share her feelings with me that I would understand. She has not been able to share or talk about her experience with me. Nor does she know that I experienced incest. Sharing this, I feel, would bring her more pain.

While growing up, I loved my biological father, but I hated his actions. As an adult I now realize he had some real problems.

I live in Arizona now, and for the last ten years my mother and stepdad have spent their winters in Arizona. So I get to visit with them when they come south from Idaho in October and when they return north in March.

Over the years, God has brought healing (a gradual process) to my life. For the last two years, the desire for a marriage relationship has been growing stronger. I know God has plans and a purpose for my life. God creates life; He is anti-death.

The Bible reference that has influenced my life a lot is Psalm 139: 13-16: "You made all the delicate inner parts of my body, and knit them together in my mother's womb. Thank you for making me so wonderfully complex. It is amazing to think about. Your workmanship is marvelous and how well I know it.

You were there while I was being formed in utter seclusion! You saw me before I was born and scheduled each day of my life before I began to breathe. Every day is recorded in your Book!"

From my own experience of incest, I would counsel a woman who was pregnant as a result of rape or incest not to have an abortion. Abortion is a means to ignore the victim, her deepest feelings of life, and her needs. It leaves destructive scars that last a lifetime.

Instead, I would share with her better options. I would encourage her to give birth to the life God is forming inside her. I would share with her how unique and special the formation of human life is inside the womb; how unique and special she is in God's eyes; that God has a plan and purpose for each life that is conceived, a very special plan; and that man is not like the other created forms of life, but is special, set apart, created in the image of God for God's honor and glory.

Human life, created by God's hand, can never be duplicated by man. We are very uniquely made—formed by God in the womb. There is only one of you. There are no duplications of you. You are unique. God made you and threw away the pattern, so to speak.

"Uniquely woman, uniquely me. That's what God made me to be."

SECTION IV

FINDING BETTER ANSWERS

CHAPTER ELEVEN

TWO WRONGS WON'T MAKE IT RIGHT: INCEST CASE EXPOSES SHORTCOMINGS OF JUDICIAL AND MEDICAL REVIEW OF ABORTION CASES

David C. Reardon, Ph.D.

In July of 1998, a Michigan judge issued a temporary restraining order blocking the parents of a 12-year-old girl from transporting her to Kansas for a late-term partial-birth abortion. The girl was 28 weeks pregnant and had allegedly been impregnated by her 17-year-old brother. She and her family had come to the United States from India about a year before and spoke little English.

Prosecutors began investigating the incest charge after receiving a tip from one of the girl's relatives, who had just learned the girl was pregnant. The girl's brother was charged with first-degree criminal sexual conduct—a felony charge that could result in life in prison and possible deportation.

Abortions after 24 weeks are banned in Michigan except to save the life of the mother. When the parents began to make arrangements for an abortion in Kansas, the prosecutor asked the judge to assume custody of the girl so she wouldn't be rushed into an abortion by her embarrassed parents.

According to newspaper reports, there were indications that the girl did not want to have an abortion. The judge issued the restraining order until the girl could undergo a psychological evaluation.

A week later, on July 24, the prosecutor asked the judge to withdraw the restraining order. He said the parents' attorneys had assured him that the girl and her parents had received counseling from experts who agreed an abortion would be in her best interests. The judge granted the prosecutor's request without hearing any testimony or cross-examination of these experts.

The girl was subsequently taken to the infamous abortionist George Tiller in Wichita where she underwent a late-term, partial birth abortion. She was about 29 weeks pregnant. Approximately 70 percent of babies born at 29 weeks gestation survive without major complications. Her child was not given this 70 percent chance to survive.

This case demonstrates three points: (1) the judicial review process doesn't work, (2) abortionists are recommending abortions despite evidence that it will not help and will almost certainly injure their patients, and (3) society has consistently failed to give incest victims the love and support they need.

PUTTING GIRLS AT RISK: NON-ADVERSARIAL PROCEEDINGS

The juvenile court system in America is woefully ill-prepared to review the question of when, if ever, abortion might be beneficial to minors. This problem exists (1) whenever the minor is a ward of the state, as in the incest case described above, or (2) whenever a minor is seeking to avoid state requirements for parental notice or consent for an abortion.

The problem is that these hearings are non-adversarial. In other words, there is no attorney representing the position that abortion is harmful and not in the girl's best interests.

In the Michigan case, the attorneys for this girl and her parents simply had to find "qualified experts" who were willing to provide sworn statements supporting the view that abortion was in her best interests.

Because there was no attorney representing the other view, these experts, their qualifications, and the medical basis for their conclusions were not subject to cross examination. Nor was the court given the opportunity to hear experts who held the opposite view—that abortion was contraindicated.

In short, the system ensures that judges hear only one side of the evidence—the pro-abortion side.

Since their rulings must be based on the preponderance of evidence presented, judges have very little leeway to refuse the recommendation of any "expert" provided by an abortion clinic. The result is that judicial bypass hearings are almost always "rubber stamp" procedures.

Without a process that provides for cross examination of witnesses and the introduction of testimony from experts who would dispute the girl's maturity or the benefit of abortion to her, judges cannot actually "judge" the evidence. Instead, the judge's role has been reduced to simply certifying that the girl's/clinic's attorneys have met the minimum threshold requirement of providing an "expert opinion" that the girl is mature or would benefit from an abortion.

The one-sided nature of such hearings has already forced at least one judge to resign from the bench. In 1995, Omaha judge Joseph Moylan asked to be excused from his first judicial bypass hearing because Nebraska's new law required that the presiding judge "shall" approve of the abortion if the preponderance of evidence supported the conclusion that the girl is mature or that the abortion would be in her best interests. Moylan's superior refused to excuse him from the case on the grounds that if one such request was granted, other judges would want out of abortion cases, too. Knowing that the evidence would all be presented from one side, and that he would be bound by the "preponderance" of that evidence, Moylan resigned rather than violate his conscience by participating in the approval of an abortion.

The solution to this problem is simple. State laws should be amended to require the courts to appoint an attorney to argue the position that (1) the abortion is contrary to the girl's best interests, (2) she is not mature enough to make this dangerous choice without her parents' knowledge, and/or (3) there is no evidence of abuse that would justify excluding the parents from being informed.

Unfortunately, at this time, no state has yet corrected this problem. In the meantime, even judges who agree that abortion is dangerous can do little to protect our teenagers from the "experts."

THE "MENTAL HEALTH" LOOPHOLE

When the Michigan story first made the headlines, pro-abortion groups immediately began to promote the notion that abortion was necessary to protect this girl's mental health, or at least to facilitate her healing from the emotional trauma of incest. It is worth noting that while many abortion advocates offered their "expert" opinions, none offered any evidence to support their claims.

Why? Because there is not one shred of evidence to support the idea that abortion ever benefits a woman's mental health even in general, much less in the specific case of an incest victim. Instead, this girl is at an extraordinary high risk of suffering severe emotional harm because of her abortion.

Listing just a few of the known risk factors for more severe post-abortion reactions clearly demonstrates that abortion was contraindicated for this girl. These risk factors include: being a teenager, having a second or third trimester abortion, having a history of mental illness or unresolved psychological trauma, being pressured to abort by others, and aborting in violation of prior moral beliefs against abortion.

Despite these risk factors, Tiller recommended a late-term abortion on the grounds that it would benefit the girl's mental health.

Tiller made this recommendation to take advantage of a "loop hole" in Kansas law that allows for late term partial-birth abortions when "continuation of the pregnancy will cause a substantial and irreversible impairment of a major physical or mental function of the pregnant woman."

Physical risks aside (and there is no evidence that childbirth would have been more dangerous to this girl than was a late-term abortion procedure) it is clear that the emotional damage associated with incest and incest pregnancy had already been done. There is no evidence that continuing the pregnancy through the last few weeks would have caused any additional "substantial" or "irreversible" emotional damage. Indeed, as will be shown below, all the evidence suggests that abortion would cause far more harm than good.

Hopefully the state attorney general will eventually force Tiller to face a grand jury and produce the medical evidence supporting his position that abortion was necessary to prevent this young girl, or any of his other late-term abortion patients, from suffering "substantial and irreversible impairment" of their mental health. It is certain that if Tiller is ever called to task, any "evidence" he produces will be long on personal opinions and bereft of *any* substantiated medical research.

IGNORING VICTIMS TO PROMOTE ABORTION

In the debate surrounding this case, it was clear that the most important voices are being drowned out by the politics of abortion. The silenced voices are those of other women who themselves became pregnant as a result of incest.

We have collected testimonies from more than two dozen such women for this book. Some placed their children for adoption. Others submitted to abortion. Of the latter, none chose abortion freely.

One 15-year-old girl was drugged and strapped to the table by an abortionist who insisted that her parents knew best. Years later, she wrote to us: "I grieve every day for my daughter. I have struggled to forget the abuse and the abortion. I can do neither. All I think of is, 'I should have done more, fought more, struggled more for the life of my child.'"

In every case we have reviewed, incest victims rejected abortion for one or all of the following reasons:

First, they saw their pregnancies as a way to expose and stop the incest.

Second, as victims of exploitation, they longed for a truly loving and non-exploitative relationship. They envisioned this hope as being fulfilled in a baby of their own whom they could love and protect.

Third, they had strong ideals about right and wrong. One of these ideas was that younger children, even unborn children, should always be protected.

Adults tend to dismiss the maternal instincts of a 12-year-old as a "playing with dolls" fantasy. But just because a 12-year-old may not be mature enough to raise a child by herself does not mean that she is incapable of loving and bonding with her preborn child.

FALSE PROMISES AND ENDLESS LIES

Incest victims grow up in a world of exploitation and deception. Yet abortion prolongs their victimization because by its very nature, it demands still more deception.

Because incest pregnancies are almost always discovered late, the unborn babies these girls are carrying are identical to the endoscopic images so popular with expectant parents: beautifully-formed babies who move their fingers, kick, cry, suck their thumbs, and peacefully sleep in the warmth of their mothers' wombs. No doubt any adult pushing a young incest victim toward an abortion would immediately agree that such pictures and films must be carefully hidden from her.

And certainly the abortionists can never honestly tell these young girls how their babies will be dismembered. Certainly Tiller didn't explain to this girl how he would suck out her child's brains before he extracted him from her womb. Such ghastly details would surely have sent her screaming from the room.

It takes a sophisticated mind, one that has mastered the philosophical arguments about choice and personhood, to justify a pragmatic choice for abortion. For girls who would have nightmares if they witnessed the killing of a deformed puppy, the thought of killing a human baby, much less *their own child*, is unfathomable.

So, they must be deceived, if only "for their own good."

But such deceptions cannot be sustained forever.

Edith Young, an incest victim who was impregnated by her stepfather when she was 12, did not understand what had happened during her abortion until she pieced the facts together during a health class three years later. The revelation knocked her over like an eighteen-wheeler. She became depressed, suicidal, and alcoholic.

"There have been a countless number of nights when I've gone without sleep just so I wouldn't dream," Edith wrote at age 37. "Often I cry. Cry because I could not stop the attacks. Cry because my daughter is dead. And I cry because it still hurts . . . . My daughter, how I miss her . . . . Even though I didn't have any say about the abortion, it has had a greater impact on my life than the rape/incest. . . . Problems are not ended by abortion, but only made worse."

All the other incest victims we interviewed vehemently expressed the same belief: *abortion made their problems worse*. Yet society continues to turn a deaf ear to their pleas. Like their parents, we want to offer them a "quick fix."

No doubt this girl's parents left Kansas feeling as though they had done something to correct an embarrassing family problem and restore their daughter's life to the way it "should be." But it was a false hope. Perhaps they have already begun to discover that it was all just a comforting lie.

Unfortunately, for the pregnant incest victim, this isn't a choice between having a baby or not having a baby. The choice is really between having a baby or having an abortion.

The latter is a frighteningly real, traumatic, life-changing event. Like the incest, it too will remain in her memory forever.

This article was originally printed in The Post-Abortion Review, *Vol. 6(3), Summer 1998. Reprinted with permission.*

CHAPTER TWELVE

FINDING REAL ANSWERS FOR PREGNANT SEXUAL ASSAULT VICTIMS

Amy R. Sobie

Kay Zibolsky is the founder of Life After Assault League, an organization dedicated to ministering to victims of sexual assault. In 1957, Kay herself was raped and became pregnant at the age of 16. She gave birth to her daughter, Robin, and placed her for adoption when she was 18 months old. Nearly 25 years later, mother and daughter were finally reunited.

The Life After Assault League (LAAL) takes a Biblical/Christian approach to counseling that is based on Kay's own experience of healing from sexual assault. The final step in this process (which involves accepting Jesus as Savior and forgiving those who have hurt you) is to "become a doer of the Word" by helping other women find healing. LAAL relies mostly on word-of-mouth to attract women, whom Kay counsels by mail, over the phone, or one-on-one locally.

We interviewed Kay for this book in order to get her perspective on sexual assault pregnancies and abortion. Kay has counseled thousands of women. (She says she lost count at about 2,000.) She believes that the occurrence of pregnancies from sexual assault is vastly under reported. According to Kay:

> About half the women I counsel are pregnant from some kind of assault. Remember that these women come from all over the world. Often times they are referred to me by pro-life groups or crisis pregnancy centers. Sometimes it is a friend or a boyfriend or a parent who calls for them.
>
> You can't say it doesn't happen. I know from my own experience that there are more rape pregnancies than the statistics say. Eighty to ninety percent of the women I have counseled who are pregnant from sexual assault have never reported the rape.

Most women Kay talks to are pregnant at the time they call her. She urges these women not to dwell on the circumstances of their baby's conception.

"People don't normally walk around thinking about how they were conceived," she said. "That's not something we dwell on. Once we're here, what does it matter how we got here?"

ABORTION IS NOT THE ANSWER

Kay said she is able to steer most of these women away from choosing abortion. She said:

Abortion is not compassionate. We think we have all the answers—we walk around making decisions for others. That baby is a human being and we have no right to make decisions for him or her. We have no right to decide someone else's life.

Abortion was not legal [when I was pregnant]—I did not know the word 'abortion.' But I do remember in the first four to six weeks wanting to get rid of the baby, wanting to beat my belly . . . or do something I had heard might cause a miscarriage. I didn't, of course, but I wanted to. I didn't want to be pregnant—I knew I would have to leave school, that people would talk . . .

But as the pregnancy progressed, as I could feel my baby begin to kick and move, my thoughts began to change. The baby itself was a part of the healing. I began to like it, even to like being pregnant. I began to know we would get through it. My mom was a single mom (my parents divorced when I was just a baby) and I knew that if she had made it, we would too.

Everyone's mind changes . . . that's why we want them to wait, to give them time to think, time for a pro-lifer to talk with them—before they do something they can't change.

You have to work with them where they are at. You have to let the Lord speak through you. Sometimes He gives you things to say that will change a woman's mind and you don't even know it.

I tell these women that there is no reason to kill a baby. I give them no loopholes. Every abortion is for someone's convenience. There are no "unwanted" children—it's just a matter of distribution. There is no reason to have an abortion—it's that simple.

Kay believes that abortion only compounds the anger women feel toward the perpetrators who attacked them. Abortion is simply a form of transferring that anger to an innocent victim.

"The rape crisis centers and secular counselors have it all

wrong when they tell the women they need to get angry so they can get over the rape," she said. "You don't need to tell a rape victim to get angry; they already are. The anger is what they need to get rid of. Otherwise they take on the guilt of the perpetrator and start hating him. Then they end up turning the anger against the baby—against the wrong person. Even if the perpetrator is caught, he is not killed for his crime of rape. Yet why do we kill the baby for the rape?"

LEARNING TO HEAL

It is holding on to this anger that prevents women from healing, Kay believes. She believes that without forgiveness for the perpetrator, there can be no true healing from the pain of sexual assault.

> I have women call who have gone to counseling for five to ten years who say they can't find healing They don't have Jesus, so they can't forgive and they can't heal. They need to realize that the counselor can't heal them.
>
> Some of the most violent cases of gang rape that I have seen, the women are the most tender, the most able to forgive and heal. There was one case where a woman's body was so torn up she had to have numerous surgeries and almost could not carry the baby to term. I've seen this several times. You would think these women would be the most angry, but they are often the most loving people. They are able to forgive and go on.
>
> I tell each woman that time marches on—as it says in Scripture, "This too will pass." I tell them I will be there for them, that I will correspond with them, that they can call me. I'll give them whatever they need to get through it. Someday they will be able to look back at this crisis and know that they got through it.
>
> Sometimes I get the chance to stay with the woman through correspondence or through seeing them at church . . . I get the chance to see them get married and have other babies. One of my friends in Australia had a rape pregnancy 11 years ago and placed the child for adoption. We still correspond and she is now married and expecting another child . . . I have the privilege of being able to look back and see where she has come from.

Kay believes that resources—having the necessary financial, physical, emotional, and spiritual support available to the women—are one of the keys to helping women chose to give birth to their children rather than give in to an abortion.

"There are more resources now than when I had my baby—more help available today where there was nothing then," she said. "We have the resources to help. Crisis pregnancy centers provide all kinds of financial and medical assistance, counseling, etc. Pro-lifers can't get weary of helping and being there for the women. We need to help them get on their feet—there aren't enough pro-lifers to mother all these women. We need to help them learn how to help themselves."

ABORTION AND DESPAIR

"If a woman has had an abortion, she needs to recognize that it was wrong; but that Jesus loves and forgives," Kay said. "She needs to accept Jesus. I always say we are in the restoration business, the business of restoring women's lives and peace. You need to have compassion—to meet these women where they are. Each case is different; you have to deal with each one differently. You can't apply the last case to the one who is coming in the door."

Abortion, Kay says, merely prolongs the hurt and trauma that is caused by sexual assault. Often women feel that they have gone "too far" to be forgiven and they just want to give up.

"Women come to me in such despair," she explained. "They feel that they've crossed a line somewhere and that they can never be forgiven. I have to tell them that Jesus always forgives."

Kay believes despair that can keep women trapped in the past and unable to accept the forgiveness and healing that is available to them. Abortion following a rape will only push them deeper into a state of despair. She believes from her experience that women who carry the child to term and experience giving life are less likely to despair and more likely to heal more quickly.

In talking about abortion, Kay emphasizes, as she has before, that giving birth to her child was part of her own healing from sexual assault. In her book *Healing Hidden Hurts*, Kay wrote:

> In talking with young women who are considering abortion, I have discovered that my life lends credibility to my words. And I say to you victims of sexual assault who may be experiencing

pressure to "take the easy way out" by the destructive means of legal abortion, "DON'T YIELD TO THAT TEMPTATION!"

For *your* Robin's sake, and for your own peace of mind, give her something far more precious than anyone else could ever give: LET HER LIVE! You'll be contributing to this world the self-less kind of love and caring we all so desperately need. And you'll find joy and fulfillment for yourself in doing it. You can take it from me—I've been there. [1]

NOTES

1. Zibolsky, Kay, *Healing Hidden Hurts* (Appleton, WI: Life After Assault League, 1995), p. 7-8.

CHAPTER THIRTEEN

HOW TO ARGUE AGAINST THE ABORTION OF CHILDREN CONCEIVED BY RAPE OR INCEST

David C. Reardon, Ph.D.

In this book, we have provided women who became pregnant from sexual assault an opportunity to be heard. Based on their experiences with both abortion and childbirth, it is clear that they stand unified in their opposition to the belief that abortion is the "best solution" to sexual assault pregnancies.

The evidence is clear. Communicating it, however, can be very difficult. This is because the misconceptions and fears surrounding sexual assault pregnancies run very deep.

In any conversation where the issue of abortion in cases of rape or incest is raised, your listeners will be inclined to judge, label, and categorize you as soon as you complete your first sentence. This is why even your first sentence must be able to open their hearts and minds to thoughtful introspection and a desire to know more. Otherwise, you will be immediately dismissed as "one of them!"

The challenge is even greater for politicians and other public figures. Their words will be limited by the media to a "sound bite" of only one or two sentences. Even a carefully explained position will be reshaped and summarized by reporters, often in very inaccurate ways. They will be quoted out of context. They will be made to look like ignorant, heartless monsters willing to "force" a woman to have "a rapist's child."

This is the trap. If you oppose abortion in cases of rape or incest, you will be accused of lacking compassion. If you accept abortion in such cases, you will be discredited in the eyes of pro-life purists and accused of lacking principle. After all, they argue, if you would allow abortion in these difficult circumstances, why not in other difficult circumstances?

This trap is reminiscent of the question put to Jesus, "Is it right to pay taxes to Caesar?" If Jesus answered "yes," He could be discredited as a collaborator with the occupation forces of Rome. If He answered "no," He could be accused before the Roman officials of inciting rebellion.

Jesus avoided this trap by first asking a better question: "Whose inscription is on this coin?" "Caesar's," they responded. "Then give to Caesar what is Caesar's and to God what is God's," Jesus replied.

Jesus' answer was both unexpected and impossible to dispute. But his answer was preceded first by his reframing the question. Before He would answer His questioners, He required them to first answer a question of His own. In this manner, He forced them to make an admission that provided not only a way out of the political trap they had devised, but also a way to refocus His listeners' minds on the spiritual imperative of following God's will.

The same approach can be applied to the question: "Do you support abortion in cases of rape or incest?"

WHERE IS YOUR COMPASSION?

Before explaining how to reframe this question, let's take a moment to look at two arguments that *don't* work.

First, many pro-lifers try to emphasize the rarity of sexual assault pregnancies. This is a weak, evasive argument. Whether few or many, sexual assault pregnancies do occur. Indeed, there is significant evidence that they may occur far more often than most people realize.[1]

This argument is generally made with the intent of pointing out that since these cases account for less than one percent of all abortions, this "hard case" issue should not dictate a public policy of abortion on request. That is true. But it is not a convincing response to the specific issue at hand.

Indeed, the argument that these cases are rare can be interpreted as lacking both compassion and principle. While pro-lifers *do* feel great compassion for women facing such a difficult situation, this argument appears to dismiss concern for the victims of a circumstance that is too "rare" to deserve public consideration. It appears to lack principle because it also implies that pro-lifers might be content to allow abortion in these "rare" cases if only the other side would agree to stop the other 99 percent. No matter how compassionate or principled the pro-lifer might be who is making this point, it is fundamentally just an argument about statistics that fails to demonstrate either one's compassion or one's principles.

The second approach is to simply and boldly assert that the right to life of the unborn child is inviolable. No matter what injuries or trauma a woman may have suffered, or may yet suffer because of her pregnancy, it does not justify the killing of an innocent human life.

As a declaration of moral principle, this answer is clear and unambiguous. But in the present situation of widespread moral confusion, which is compounded by a nearly universal ignorance of the truth about both abortion and sexual assault pregnancies, this answer *appears* to lack compassion.

I must emphasize that this is a defect in appearance only. God's moral law is given to us for the purpose of helping us find good and avoid evil. From the Christian world view, it is easy to anticipate and see that the right moral choices lead to the best possible long-range results. Bad moral choices may bring temporary benefit but lead to long-term problems. Therefore, if we desire good for others we will encourage them to make the right moral decision in every circumstance, regardless of the short-term consequences.

Such advice does not lack compassion. Instead, it reflects a spiritually *informed compassion*. It is a compassion that desires the best for another person over the long term, both on earth and for eternity.

The problem is that we no longer live in a society that automatically sees *informed compassion* in statements of moral principle. Indeed, most modern Americans have been robbed of their belief in the existence of moral absolutes.

We must recognize that the prevailing ethic is pragmatism. Acts like abortion, which many pragmatists might admit to be immoral if used for "selfish" reasons, is tolerated, accepted, and even recommended in the "hard cases" where it *appears* to be beneficial or necessary in the name of "compassion."

Because they have lost sight of God's moral law (which is an expression of love and unchanging absolute truths), pragmatists are blind to the compassion of those who preach moral absolutes. This is why people who oppose abortion, especially in cases of rape and incest, are not respected as idealists but are instead scorned as heartless, rigid and judgmental.

The solution is to reframe the question in such a way that even moral pragmatists can understand and agree with the answer.

THE SOLUTION

When Jesus answered the question about the Roman tax, He shifted the question from one of politics and morality to one of ownership: "Give to Caesar what is Caesar's, and to God what is God's."

On the surface, his answer is simple and pragmatic. On further reflection, however, it leaves unresolved the question of what belongs to Caesar and what to God. After all, everything that was Caesar's was also God's. In addition, the direction to give the coin to Caesar could have two meanings; either simply "Pay the tax," or, "The use of this Roman coin is itself a collaboration with the occupying force and puts you under Caesar's rule. Give it back to Caesar if you want to be free of Caesar. Give yourself only to God." In addition, while Christ's answer hints at moral questions of both civil and religious obedience, He did not use that opportunity to go into a long exhortation about how we can resolve or balance our obedience to conflicting civil and religious duties.

My point here is that Jesus did not attempt to completely resolve every aspect of the question posed to Him. His immediate purpose was two fold: first, to expose His questioners' hypocrisy (by asking them to hold forth one of Caesar's coins that they carried in their purses), and second, to escape their attempt to force Him into the mold of either a collaborator or an insurrectionist. He accomplished these goals by giving an honest, practical answer, but not an answer that would resolve every possible permutation of the question that was raised. Indeed, if the scribes had pressed Jesus further, it is likely that He would have again responded with questions of His own. If they had refused to answer His questions, He might then have refused to answer theirs (Mk 11:28-33).

With this in mind, I believe pro-life Christians must address the question of abortion for rape and incest with both honesty and cunning. There are times and places when one might be able to fully explain why abortion in sexual assault cases is never right, both for moral reasons and because it will only hurt the women we want to help. Such cases exist when one is addressing a non-hostile, pro-life audience or when one has ample opportunity to lay out a substantial body of evidence, such as in a lengthy magazine article.

But in most circumstances when this question is raised in a public or private discussion, it is raised with the intent of forcing the pro-life advocate to choose between being labeled either heartless or unprincipled. In such cases, it is imprudent and impractical to lay out the complete case against abortion in these "hard cases." Instead, one should have more limited goals: (1) to avoid being labeled and dismissed; (2) to express our concern for and solidarity with women in this situation; and (3) to challenge one's listeners to think and probe more deeply into the question of what *really* is most beneficial to women in these difficult circumstances.

To demonstrate how this can be done, I have written below an exchange between a hard-core pro-abortion reporter and "Jane," an imaginary pro-life political candidate making her first bid for elective office.

This is one of the most difficult circumstances imaginable. Jane is on record as being a pro-life candidate, and she knows the reporter is looking for any opportunity to misrepresent her as being either a heartless ideologue or a pandering compromiser. She wants to be honest in every answer, but at the same time she wants to deprive the reporter of the opportunity to label her as heartless and rigid.

In preparing for her campaign, Jane has not only read *Victims and Victors,* she has also read *Making Abortion Rare: A Healing Strategy for a Divided Nation* (Springfield, IL: Acorn Books, 1996 . . . plug, plug.) This has prepared her to articulate a very pro-woman view on abortion in general. She has a position statement on record regarding her goal to protect women from dangerous and unwanted abortions by making abortion clinics more fully liable for any physical or psychological injuries that may result from an abortion. She believes that the well-being of the mother and child is always intertwined and that abortion is inherently dangerous and never medically justified. By focusing her answers on her desire to protect women, she knows that her proposals will also protect unborn children.

At first glance, some people may consider Jane's responses to be evasive. This is especially true of those who simply want clear-cut, blunt answers like, "I oppose abortion in every circumstance." The problem with such answers, however, is that they invite labeling and let the reporter control the conversation to suit his own ends. While Jane should clearly articulate her opposition to abortion with pro-lifers (for example, on pro-life "scorecards" that ask candidates to indicate their position on various pro-life issues), she should try to avoid making statements that could be used by pro-abortion reporters to paint her as an "anti-choice radical" who doesn't care about women.

You may also note this irony. The reporter, who represents the moral relativists, is consistently trying to pin Jane down to an absolutist moral position so he can portray her as "closed-minded." He, who has no firm moral principles, is mostly interested in her moral views so that he can "expose" her moral rigidity. On the other hand, Jane, who has moral principles, prefers to focus her answers on the *scientific fact* that abortion hurts women (which is the automatic byproduct of a bad moral choice.) This is not a betrayal of her moral beliefs. It is instead an insistence on conveying her moral beliefs in a manner that can best influence the opinions of pragmatists.

HOLDING THE LINE—IN SOUND BITES

Reporter: What is your position on abortion?

Jane: I believe we absolutely must protect the right of women to be fully informed about the risks of abortion and their right to get good, qualified medical advice. And we also need to pass laws that will make it easier for women to recover damages for the physical and psychological injuries that can result from an abortion. Too many abortion clinics are now operating at a dangerously poor level of care.

Reporter: Would you support legislation that would limit a woman's right to have an abortion?

Jane: I want to sponsor and support legislation that protects women. I would hope that legislators on all sides of this issue will join me in my effort to pass a law that will protect women from being pressured into *unwanted* abortions by other people, whether that pressure comes from boyfriends, parents, husbands, school counselors, or physicians.

Reporter: But do you think abortion should be legal?

Jane: I don't believe the state should ever sanction the killing of innocent human beings. But as a legislator, I have no control over the legal status of abortion. The courts have made it legal. On the other hand, the courts have failed to make abortion safe. Until the question of legality is returned to the legislature, all I can do is to try to protect women's interests as much as I can.

Reporter: Do you support abortion in cases of rape or incest?

Jane: Women who are victims of rape or incest deserve just as much care as other women. Indeed, they deserve even better and more extensive screening and counseling than the average woman faced with an unplanned pregnancy. I don't see how it can be of any benefit to them if they are rushed into an abortion, regardless of the risks, simply because they have been assaulted. That would only risk victimizing them a second time.

Reporter: But do you think it is morally right to provide abortions in such cases?

Jane: Isn't the real question about how we can best help these women? Do you think abortion benefits these women?

Reporter: Well, I wouldn't want to have a rapist's baby.

Jane: Of course not. No one wants to be raped. But the question is whether or not the abortion will make the woman's life better or worse. Isn't that what we should really be concerned about?

Reporter: Well, of course it makes their lives better. They aren't stuck with a child that's a constant reminder of their attacker.

Jane: That's what many people presume. But I have read the testimonies of women who have had sexual assault pregnancies, including a book that presents the views of nearly 200 such women. Those who carried to term said that process of going through the pregnancy and giving birth to their child actually helped to heal from the sexual assault by helping to restore their sense of self-worth. Likewise, many of those who had abortions said the abortion was harder to deal with than the rape or incest. I've read many of these testimonies myself. On the other hand, I have yet to see one medical or psychological study that shows any benefit from abortion in these cases. After seeing all this evidence, it just isn't clear to me that abortion is the best option in these difficult cases.

Reporter: So you oppose abortion in cases of rape or incest?

Jane: I'm still trying to develop an informed opinion. Like you, I simply want to see these women helped in the best way possible. If there is evidence that abortion will be helpful, this should be presented to the woman and her doctors who have a duty to protect her health. If there is evidence that it will be harmful, this too should be presented to the woman. And if a doctor recommends an abortion, in this or any circumstance, when abortion may actually be contraindicated, he should be held liable.

Reporter: Would you vote against government funding of abortions in cases of rape or incest?

Jane: Again, I think funding should be determined by whether or not it can be shown that this would actually benefit women. I don't think the funding issue can be responsibly addressed without first having legislative hearings where we would invite these women to speak for themselves. We need to hear directly from women who have been pregnant as a result of sexual assault, not just from abortion advocates who claim to be speaking on their behalf. We shouldn't be basing this decision on preconceptions or on a political agenda to promote public acceptance of abortion in general. Without such hearings, we would really be voting only on the basis of our preconceptions or ideology. These women deserve a chance to be heard. If we are too hasty and choose to fund something that may actually hurt women, I think that would be negligent on our part.

Reporter: You talk about making abortion providers more liable for abortion-related injuries. Aren't your proposals actually intended to drive doctors out of business and make it more difficult for women to get abortions, regardless of their circumstances?

Jane: If abortion is as safe as abortion providers have been telling us, tough liability standards will simply keep away the "medical hacks." I would think both pro-choice and pro-life people would be glad about that. But also, my proposal is simply to codify the high professional standard of care which the Supreme Court envisioned and described in *Roe v. Wade* and other cases. It is the obligation of the physician to make an informed and responsible medical recommendation to the woman and to ensure that a woman's choice to abort is fully informed and in her best interests. I don't see how anyone who truly cares about the rights and safety of women could oppose my proposal, that simply makes it easier for these women to recover the costs of medical care for the injuries they may suffer. The question facing legislators is really to decide which is most important: protecting the health of women, or protecting the profits of abortion providers. I choose to stand on the side of women.

Reporter: But family planning advocates say that if your proposal becomes law, doctors will refuse to perform abortions because of the increased liability risk.

Jane: If abortion is as safe as they claim, then women won't sue and juries won't grant any damages. The only reason these doctors would stop doing abortions is if they believed that abortion causes more injuries than they have been telling us, or those particular doctors are merely the worst in the field and most likely to be sued. Look, abortion providers have opposed every form of state regulation of their business. They want this to be simply something between women and their doctors. In that case, we should at least allow women to regulate the standards of the abortion industry through civil liability. By making it easier for women to enforce liability we are protecting women by discouraging low quality care at abortion clinics. What could be more pro-woman than that?

THE IMPORTANCE OF LEGISLATIVE HEARINGS

In the preceding exchange, Jane addressed the issue of rape and incest pregnancies in the context of a larger agenda to protect the health and well being of women. While avoiding a direct attack on the abortion industry, which would then put her in the position of having to prove her charges (a time consuming task), she simply conveys a sense of suspicion about the motives and standard of care within the abortion industry. On the specific question of abortion for children conceived in rape, she clearly indicates her doubts that abortion is beneficial and expresses her desire to hold hearings that would allow women who have actually had sexual assault pregnancies to speak out on their own behalf.

This call for hearings should be an important part of the pro-life legislators' response to this issue. The public is ignorant of the evidence presented in this book. A flat-out statement of opposition to abortion in these cases undermines the public's perception that the pro-life legislator is reasonable and compassionate. A call for hearings so these women can speak out for themselves, on the other hand, adds to the legislators' image of being reasonable and compassionate. Hearings provide a process by which the public can be educated. They provide a basis for legislators to make decisions based on *informed compassion*.

Pro-life politicians often make the defense of the child's rights the primary focus of their arguments against abortion. While this is admirable, it is a strategic mistake because most politicians are simply not the best spokespersons for the unborn. It is the women who have lost their children to abortion who are the best possible spokespersons for their children. It is their testimonies that most accurately reflect the truth about abortion and about the sanctity of unborn children. Politicians would be much more effective in their pro-life efforts if they would concentrate their efforts on giving these women a platform to speak out and by using their influence to insist that the public should listen to these testimonies.

Political or moral arguments are not the principal way in which public perceptions and attitudes are changed. The most effective tool for changing public opinion is the story. Harriet Beecher Stowe's *Uncle Tom's Cabin* is proof of that. Abraham Lincoln himself credited her story with having awakened a nation to the horror of slavery. The awakening was so profound it culminated in the Civil War.

In the case of abortion, I am firmly convinced that it is the stories of the women and men who chose abortion and have suffered so much from that dreadful mistake that are the key to changing the general public's attitudes about abortion. Through their stories, we hear that these women and men did not lose "products of conception"; they lost their *children*. When we hear their stories—either directly or as relayed to us by politicians, pro-life advocates, or in the media—we become witnesses to the emotional connection between women and the children they have aborted. These stories will convert minds and hearts far more effectively than political arguments or moral reasoning.

Consider, for example, the testimonies contained in these pages. Whether they carried the child to term or had an abortion, these women have born powerful witness to the sacredness of their children's lives. They have spoken eloquently about how offering abortion in such cases is a dangerous temptation that leads to far more harm than good. And through the children who escaped abortion, the world sees the joy and pride of mothers who once wept. Without these stories, it is impossible to make a compelling case against abortion—especially in the "hard cases."

This is why legislative hearings are so important. They provide a forum for women who have actually been in the situation of being pregnant by sexual assault to tell their stories. Such hearings should not be limited to "experts." Only the women who have actually become pregnant by sexual assault are *truly* qualified to testify about this complex experience. Many of the 192 women who contributed information to our study have expressed a willingness to participate in such hearings.

In light of the testimonies and survey findings described in this book, the burden of proving that abortion is a good choice in these cases should fall on the pro-abortionists. Legislators should demand that they support their view by bringing forward the authentic testimony of women who became pregnant through sexual assault and who either (1) benefitted from abortion or (2) suffered from being "forced" to carry their children to term.

Any such testimony, if it exists at all, should then be weighed to compare the women's testimony from both sides regarding the harm of having an abortion versus the harm of being "forced" to carry to term, and the benefits of carrying to term versus the presumed benefits of having an abortion. In making this evaluation, the testimony of women who aborted a child conceived during sexual assault should also be evaluated in light of the finding that the average period of time that lapses before women become aware of abortion-related emotional problems is eight to ten years.

In addition, it should be noted that the testimony of sexual assault victims who did *not* become pregnant is irrelevant to the question of whether or not abortion is appropriate in these cases. Such women, who can be found in every walk of life and among every political persuasion, can only speak about their own fears, angers, and expectations *if* they had conceived a child. But they did not, perhaps because in God's mercy, He knew this was not a cross they could bear. While their testimony about the experience of sexual assault would be valid, they simply have no experience from which to speak about pregnancy resulting from sexual assault.

NOTES

1. Melisa M. Holmes, et.al., "Rape-related Pregnancies: Estimates and Descriptive Characteristics from a National Study of Women" *Am J Obstet Gynecol* 175(2): 320-324, August 1996. In this study based on a survey of approximately 4000 women, the researchers estimated that there may be as many as 32,000 pregnancies each year resulting from acts of sexual assault, with approximately half of these among women under 18 years of age.

AFTERWORD

It is our prayer that this collection of first-hand accounts from women who have experienced sexual assault pregnancies, the optimistic witness of children conceived through sexual assault, and the expert testimony of counselors who have worked with these victims, will help to destroy the social prejudices which irrationally embrace abortion for these "hard cases."

As we have seen, all of the existing evidence suggests that a history of sexual assault is a *contraindication* for abortion. No *informed and conscientious* physician would ever recommend abortion in these cases, since the "treatment" is clearly more likely to hurt the woman than to benefit her.

As G.K. Chesterton once observed, "Morality is like art; somewhere you have to draw a line." With regard to the issue of abortion, the only clear and justifiable place to draw the line is on the side of life, forbidding the intentional destruction of innocent life for any reason.

What is the purpose of law, except to draw lines? Indeed, if we value moral virtue, then the goal of society should be to help people become good and virtuous.

In this context, laws against abortion are not punitive; they are protective. They are intended not only to protect innocent children, but also to protect the mothers and fathers who would, in a moment of despair, otherwise consent to the slaying of their children.

Good laws reflect clear and deep thought, consideration of right and wrong, and examination of future consequences as seen in the calm light of day. Good laws are sincerely meant to guide and protect people from making errors of judgment which are objectively wrong. Laws that prohibit abortion are just such laws. They protect women and children from a deadly mistake that is usually committed in the darkness of despair, the confusion of uncertainty, and the allure of the shallow, seductive "quick-fix" mentality.

As a society we are called upon to recognize the simple fact that the welfare of a mother and her child are intimately intertwined. One can never hurt a child without hurting the child's mother. This is true both before and after the child is born. The physical, emotional, and spiritual bond is simply too intimate to be torn away without doing violence to both the mother and her child.

This is why abortion is inherently dangerous. The mother's body is designed to protect and nurture her child. Abortion breeches these defenses to destroy the child, and so must do violence to the woman's body that can result in permanent injury.

Likewise, the woman's mind and spirit are designed to develop a maternal bond of love with her child. While the child's body may be ripped from her womb, there is no way to rip the memory of her child out of her mind or the unfulfilled love for her child out of her heart. This is why the psychological, emotional, and spiritual aftereffects of abortion can never be controlled or erased. The bond between mother and child is simply too intertwined. When ever one hurts a child, born or unborn, one will also be hurting the child's mother.

There is yet another side to this truth; one cannot help a child without also helping the child's mother. Pro-life advocates must continue to vigorously respond to this truth, demonstrating our commitment to serve women faced with problem pregnancies in ever more loving and sacrificial ways.

In the end, our goal is not simply to make abortion illegal. Our goal is to make it *unthinkable*. This requires three steps.

First, we must educate women, men, and their families about the severe and lasting negative effects of abortion on women.

Second, we must begin to hold abortionists and those who encourage abortion fully liable for the injuries to women that will inevitably occur. To this end, we must make it far easier for women injured by abortion to obtain actual and punitive damages in civil courts for both the injuries they have suffered and the indignity of being exploited, lied to, and recklessly exposed to the dangers of abortion.

Third, we must create a loving, pro-life society in which every child, no matter how he or she is conceived, is welcomed and supported by family, friends, and society.

It is easy to give birth to a child when there is a thunderous applause of approval, ample resources, and ready hands to help. It is only when a woman is faced with disapproval, lack of support, and threats of isolation that the thought of giving birth to a new life—an extension of herself—becomes clouded with despair.

To create such a society—where no rational person would ever consider, much less desire, an abortion—is no easy task.

But it is a worthy goal. After all, the problem is not that women lack the desire to do what is right. The problem is that we, as a society, lack the will and commitment to help them.

AN OUTLINE OF ARGUMENTS AGAINST ABORTION IN THE "HARD CASES"

In most situations, pro-life advocates will not be in a position to fully explain the arguments against abortion in cases of sexual assault. In such cases, to simply raise doubts about whether or not abortion is actually beneficial in these circumstances is a major victory. That should be your primary goal in the few minutes you have to state your case.

In circumstances where the pro-life advocate has an opportunity to lay out a more complete argument, the following outline of points may be helpful. Together with detailed evidence and excerpts from the testimonies described earlier in this book, the pro-life position can be powerfully and successfully defended.

OUTLINE OF ARGUMENTS

I. The idea that abortion as the best solution in sexual assault pregnancies arises from prejudice against rape and incest victims.

A. Most sexual assault victims do not want abortions. Even when abortion is legal, up to 70 percent of women pregnant from rape choose to carry their pregnancies to term.

B. Frequently, rape and incest victims who do have abortions do so only under pressure from others. This occurs because of widespread misunderstanding and prejudices against rape and incest victims.

   1. Rape victims feel pressured to have an abortion to get rid of the "stain" of rape, which makes others feel uncomfortable with them.

   2. Incest victims especially are almost always forced into unwanted abortions by family members wanting to cover

up the crime. Abortion only hides the family's dysfunctions and furthers the victim's exploitation.

C. Rape and incest victims who do have abortions suffer additional psychological harm due to the abortion. Abortion lowers self-esteem and increases feelings of being violated, dirty, and guilty, which can lead to suicidal behavior, drug and alcohol abuse, sexual dysfunction, difficulties in later relationships and many other emotional and behavioral problems.

D. There is no documented evidence that rape and incest victims ever benefit from abortion. There *is* documented evidence that abortion for rape and incest victims actually make their problems worse.

II. Legalization of abortion for cases of rape and incest and funding of such abortions will increase the chances that victims will be coerced into unwanted abortions.

A. Rape and incest victims are frequently pressured into abortion by others. For the victim's friends and family, hiding the problem by a quick abortion is the best way to avoid becoming entangled in understanding and supporting the victim's real needs.

B. Legalization and/or funding of abortions for rape and incest victims adds government authority to the false idea that rape and incest pregnancies *ought* to be aborted.

C. The attitude that rape and incest victims *should* have abortions is paternalistic. Because these "paternalists" know better than the victims, undue pressure is brought to bear on pregnant victims to accept unwanted abortions.

   1. This pressure may cause a woman who has pro-life convictions to betray her own values and thus be subjected to even greater guilt.

   2. This pressure frequently makes the victim feel she has "no choice" but to undergo an abortion. Because she never truly comes to terms with the decision on her own, she is at greater risk of post-abortion trauma.

   3. Legalization and government funding for abortion sends the inaccurate message that the government has officially determined that abortion will help rape and incest vic-

tims.

III. We should be suspicious of the claims of those who use the case of pregnancy resulting from rape and incest as an example of why abortion should be legalized in all circumstances.

A. Pro-abortionists are exploiting the emotional horror, misconceptions, and prejudices of the public against rape and incest victims in order to sell the idea that abortion is necessary and beneficial in certain "hard" circumstances.

B. In fact, these "hard" cases are the "worst" cases for abortion, because abortion in these cases does even more psychological harm to women than abortion under less difficult circumstances.

C. In their efforts to promote their own social agenda, pro-abortionists have ignored the real needs and experience of rape and incest victims. They pretend to speak on their behalf for the "need" for abortion, but they do so without any authorization from sexual assault victims.

IV. The testimony of women who became pregnant through sexual assault is virtually unanimous in opposition to accepting abortion as the "best thing to do" in these circumstances.

A. Of the 56 testimonies collected in our sample of women who aborted sexual assault pregnancies, *the vast majority* (83 percent) report that the abortion only compounded their problems, and that they regret having had the abortion. The other women were either unclear as to how they felt about the abortion or stated that it was the "best possible decision" under the circumstances, although most reported some regrets or doubts about their decision. Only *one* woman stated that she had no regrets about her abortion.

B. Of the 133 testimonies collected of sexual assault victims who carried the child to term, *none* report regrets about giving birth to their children or a wish that they had chosen abortion instead. Nearly all the women report joy and healing connected with the birth of their child.

C. It is the burden of those advocating abortion as a medical "treatment" for sexual assault pregnancies to prove that there is a measurable benefit that outweighs the physical and psychological risks of the "treatment." This has not been done. Instead, the existing evidence shows that abortion is contraindicated in these circumstances.

V. It is never appropriate for the law to sanction the direct killing of an innocent human life.

  A. If there is any circumstance in which there is a sound medical basis for believing that a woman's life would be gravely endangered without an abortion, the doctor should not be subject to criminal prosecution for saving the woman's life. But such exceptions, if they ever occur, should not be sanctioned by the law but instead, should simply not be prosecuted.

  B. Clemency from prosecution should be granted only when:

    1. There was some reasonable (if not irrefutable) basis for believing the woman would die without an abortion, and

    2. The doctor and hospital did not accept any payment for this life-saving abortion. Money corrupts judgments.

ABOUT THE EDITORS

David C. Reardon, Ph.D., is a biomedical ethicist, researcher, director of the Elliot Institute for Social Sciences Research, and editor of *The Post-Abortion Review*. He has been involved in post-abortion research and education since 1983 and is considered a leading expert on post-abortion issues.

Dr. Reardon is a frequent guest on Christian radio and television talk shows and has been a keynote speaker at many state and national conventions for pro-life organizations. His previous related works include *Aborted Women, Silent No More; Making Abortion Rare: A Healing Strategy for a Divided Nation;* and *The Jericho Plan: Breaking Down the Walls Which Prevent Post-Abortion Healing*.

Julie Makimaa was conceived in rape, raised in an adoptive home, and reunited with her birth mother in 1985. Thankful for the sacrifices of her adoptive parents and birth mother, Julie shares her personal story to encourage others to recognize the tremendous value of every life.

In 1989 Julie founded Fortress International, an organization dedicated to offering support and encouragement to women who have experienced sexual assault pregnancies and children conceived in rape or incest. She has testified before a number of state legislatures, lobbied Congress and appeared on numerous radio and television talk shows, including *Donahue, Geraldo* and *Sally Jesse Raphael*. Her story has appeared in many national newspapers and magazines, including *The Los Angeles Times, The Washington Times* and *Glamour*.

In addition, Julie is the Life Issues Advocate for Family Research Council, promoting grassroots education in the areas of sanctity of life, abstinence, American heritage, citizenship and the political process. She also continues to challenge the necessity for abortion in cases of rape and incest by publicly sharing her personal story.

Amy Sobie is assistant to Dr. Reardon at the Elliot Institute and Assistant Editor of *The Post-Abortion Review*. She is a graduate of Franciscan University of Steubenville in Ohio, where she studied communications and human life issues, an extensive program examining the moral, legal, social and ethical aspects of abortion, euthanasia and other life issues. She has been active in the pro-life movement since 1993 and previously worked as a fundraising manager for Right to Life of Michigan.

How can you help others—or yourself—find emotional and spiritual healing after abortion?

Read this book!

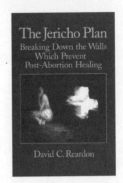

The Jericho Plan:
*Breaking Down the Walls
Which Prevent
Post-Abortion Healing*

The Jericho Plan shows how women and men struggling with past abortions feel trapped, unable to express their pain or seek comfort from their loved ones. On the one hand, they fear that those who are pro-life will condemn and reject them. On the other hand, they fear that those who are pro-choice will deny their need to grieve their loss.

Prepared with the help of experienced post-abortion counselors and clergy, *The Jericho Plan* teaches readers how to break through these and many other obstacles which prevent post-abortion healing. You will find comfort and direction for your church, your loved ones, and perhaps even yourself.

- *Learn seven steps to post-abortion healing.*

- *Become a "stealth healer" and give hope to women and men plagued by post-abortion grief—even if their abortions are still secret!*

- *Create a healing environment in your church and community by offering dynamic examples of God's mercy and grace.*

- *And much more . . .*

While useful for anyone interested in post-abortion healing, *The Jericho Plan* is especially directed toward ministers and clergy. Through background information on post-abortion issues, compelling testimonies, sample sermons, and an extensive directory of resources, it shows them how to preach on abortion in a compassionate and unifying way.

List Price: $8.95. Quantity Discounts Available.
Available through Acorn Books at **1-888-41-ACORN.**

Finally, something new to say about abortion.

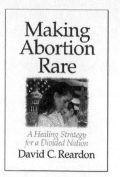

Making Abortion Rare

A Healing Strategy for a Divided Nation

David C. Reardon

Making Abortion Rare

A Healing Strategy for a Divided Nation

Is it possible for abortion to become rare even though it remains legal? Yes! This book shows readers a clear and practical strategy for making abortion not simply illegal, but unthinkable.

Making Abortion Rare reveals a comprehensive and compassionate program of pastoral, political, and educational reform that will reduce antagonism, create a healing environment for those who have been wounded by abortion, and draw Americans together through their common concern for women.

Here's what the reviewers are saying:

The Post-Abortion Review

Discount Schedule for

Victims and Victors

*Speaking Out About their Pregnancies,
Abortions and Children Resulting from Sexual Assault*

Suggested Retail Price: $11.95

# of Copies	Discount	# of Copies	Discount
1-2	none	1000-1,999	56%
3-6	20%	2000-4,999	58%
7-49	40%	5000-9,999	60%
50-99	45%	10,000-24,999	63%
100-499	50%	25,000-50,000	65%
500-1000	53%	50,000-99,999	68%
1000-1,999	56%	100,000 up	70%

Shipping & Handling*
1 book	$3.50
2 books	$6
Over 3	actual shipping costs

To Order, call Acorn Books at 1-888-41-ACORN. Credit card orders accepted.

Send purchase orders to: Acorn Books, PO Box 7348, Springfield, IL 62791.

Acorn Books is the publishing arm of the Elliot Institute, a 501(c)3 tax exempt organization. For more information about the Elliot Institute and its resources, visit the Elliot Institute web site at www.afterabortion.org. Donations to support our work are tax-deductible.

Elliot Institute
PO Box 7348
Springfield, IL 62791-7348
(217) 525-8202

*Shipping and handling prices listed here are for regular UPS shipping within the continental United States only. For information about shipping prices for other shipping methods or outside the continental U.S., call the Acorn Books order line.